Anatomy Student's Color-In Handbook

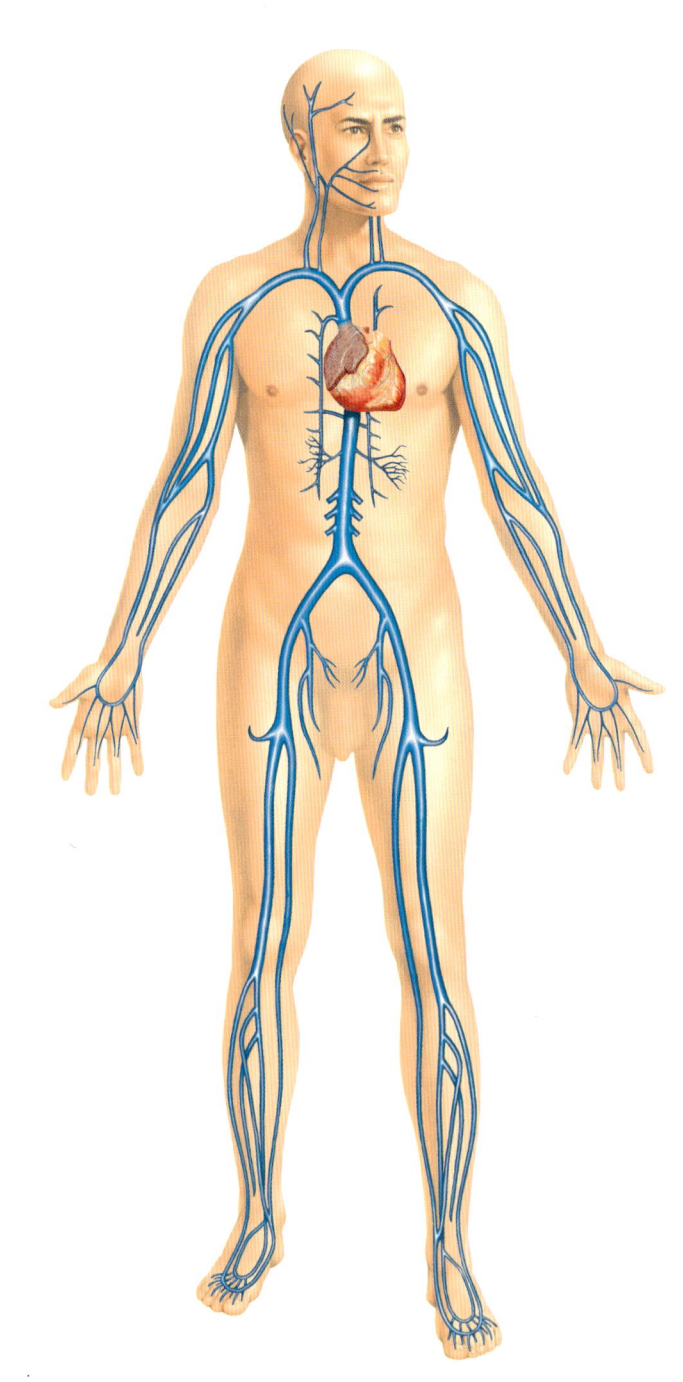

Anatomy Student's Color-In Handbook

VOLUME THREE:

Endocrine System • Circulatory System
Lymphatic System • Respiratory System

Professor Ken Ashwell, BMedSc, MBBS, PhD

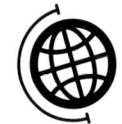

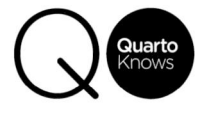

Quarto is the authority on a wide range of topics.

Quarto educates, entertains and enriches the lives of our readers—enthusiasts and lovers of hands-on living.

www.QuartoKnows.com

First published in 2017 by
Global Book Publishing Pty Ltd
Part of The Quarto Group
Level One, Ovest House,
58 West Street, Brighton, BN1 2RA, UK

ISBN: 978-0-85762-514-4

A Global Book

Printed and bound in China

Conceived, designed and produced by Global Book Publishing

Consultant Editor: Professor Ken Ashwell, BMedSc, MBBS, PhD

Designer: Angela English

Project Editor: Kathleen Steeden

Illustrations:
Joanna Culley, BA(Hons) RMIP, MMAA, IMI (Medical-Artist.com), Mike Gorman, Thomson Digital, Glen Vause

Contributors:
Robin Arnold, MSc, Ken Ashwell, BMedSc, MB, BS, PhD, Deborah Bryce, BSc, MScQual, MChiro, GrCertHEd, John Gallo, MB, BS(Hons), FRACP, FRCPA, Rakesh Kumar, MB, BS, PhD, Peter Lavelle, MB, BS, Karen McGhee, BSc, Michael Roberts, MB, BS, LLB(Hons), Emeritus Professor Frederick Rost, BSc(Med), MB, BS, PhD, DCP(London), DipRMS, Elizabeth Tancred, BSc, PhD, Dzung Vu, MD, MB, BS, DipAnat, GradCertHEd, Phil Waite, BSc(Hons), MBChB, CertHEd, PhD

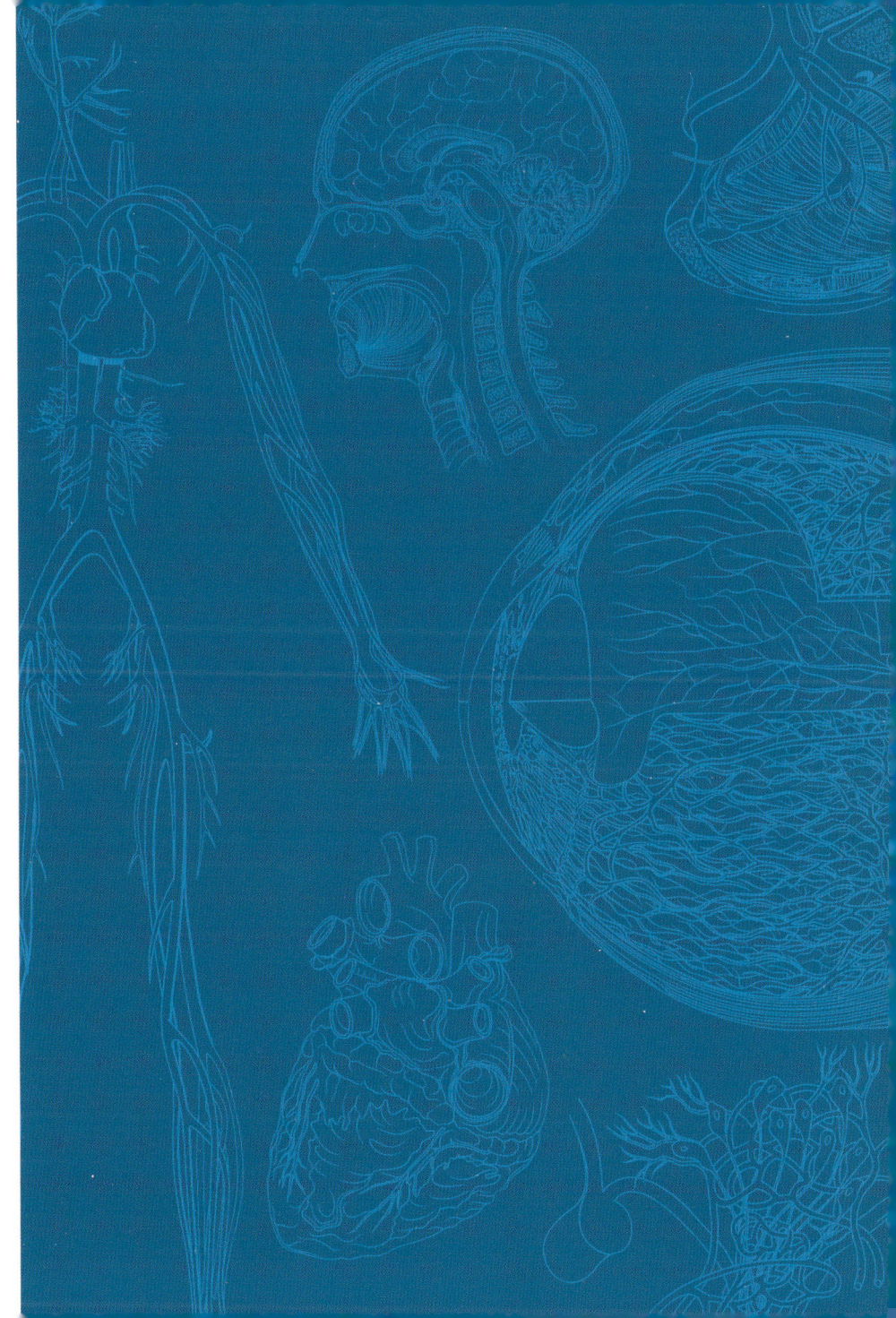

Contents

Lymphatic System

Respiratory System

Introduction

There are two important principles embodied in this book. The first is that anatomy is a three-dimensional, fundamentally visual subject, which is best learned by the student using their hand and eye to follow the position, contours, and courses of bones, muscles, vessels, and nerves. Anatomy cannot be learned simply as textual information—for proper understanding of the structure of the human body, students must be able to hold the positions, relationships, and trajectories of anatomical structures in their "mind's eye."

The second is that learning in any field, but especially in anatomy, is most effective when it is an active process. Retention of knowledge is more complete when the student is actively involved in testing themselves against the body of knowledge they wish to retain. Passive immersion in a body of information by reading text will rarely lead to any significant retention of knowledge.

By combining these two important educational principles, this book provides an effective, convenient tool for students to master the important elements of human structure. Students are encouraged to use the book in conjunction with their recommended text to absorb and reinforce critically important concepts in the topography of the human body.

Ken Ashwell, BMedSc, MB, BS, PhD
Professor of Anatomy,
Department of Anatomy,
School of Medical Sciences,
The University of New South Wales
Sydney, Australia

This book is designed to assist students and professionals to identify body parts and structures, and the numbered leader lines aid the process by clearly pointing out each body part. The function of coloring allows you to familiarize yourself with individual parts of the body and check your knowledge.

Coloring is best done using either pencils or pens in a variety of dark and light colors. Where possible, you should use the same color for like structures, so that all completed illustrations can be utilized later as visual references. According to anatomical convention, the color green is usually reserved for lymphatic structures, yellow for nerves, red for arteries, and blue for veins.

The numbered leader lines that point to separate parts of the illustration enable you to consolidate and then check your knowledge using the keys and descriptions on the facing page.

Endocrine System

The cells of the body communicate with each other by the movement of messenger chemicals called hormones. Hormones may be short or long chains of amino acids (peptides or proteins), or steroid molecules made from cholesterol. These messenger chemicals are made by specialized organs (glands) of the endocrine system and carried around the body by the bloodstream or diffused through the fluid of body cavities. Endocrine glands include the pituitary (often called the master endocrine gland), thyroid, parathyroid, thymus, adrenal, pancreatic islets, testes, and ovaries. The endocrine system produces changes in body function over periods of hours to years.

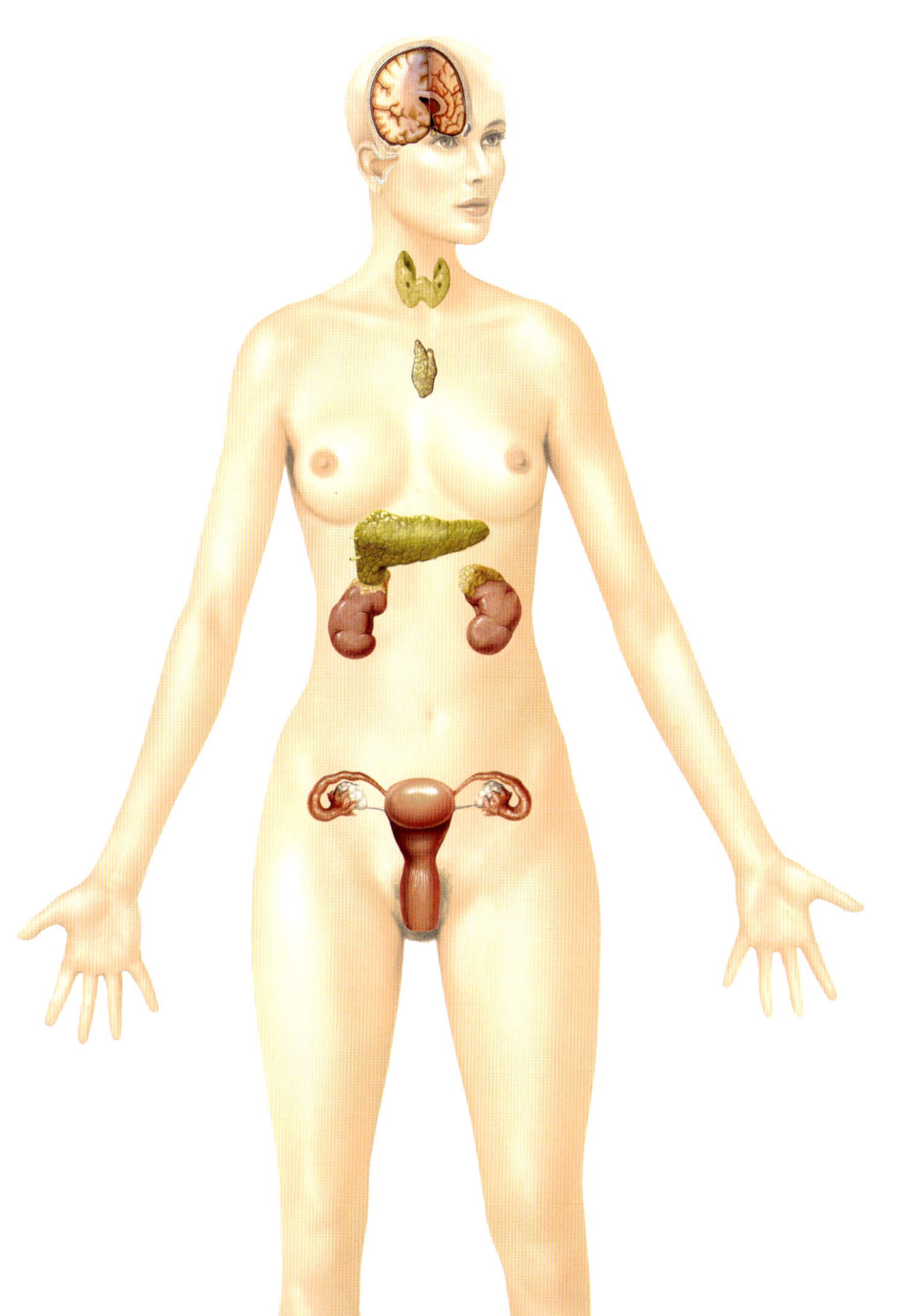

Endocrine System: Male

Key:

1 Pituitary gland
2 Parathyroid gland (on back of thyroid gland lobe)
3 Thymus gland (atrophic in adults)
4 Pancreas
5 Testes
6 Adrenal glands (includes cortex and medulla)
7 Thyroid gland
8 Pineal gland

Description:

The endocrine system, involved in coordinating the activities of tissues throughout the body, acts by means of hormones. Hormones, made of amino acids or steroids, are released from endocrine cells at specific times and in precise amounts to act on target organs. Hormones usually act by binding with special receptor sites on, or inside, target cells. Endocrine organs (often called endocrine glands) secrete mainly into the bloodstream.

Endocrine hormones affect the nervous system, and many endocrine organs are stimulated or inhibited by nerve cells. The hypothalamus of the brain has an intimate connection with the chief organ of the endocrine system, the pituitary. This means that the endocrine and nervous systems share control of body functions—the nervous system usually controls activities occurring rapidly or in the short term, while the endocrine system controls slow or long-term changes.

The organs involved in the male endocrine system are the pituitary, pineal, thymus, thyroid, parathyroids, adrenals, pancreatic islets, and testes. The testes produce hormones that control sexual function and secondary sexual characteristics.

anterior view

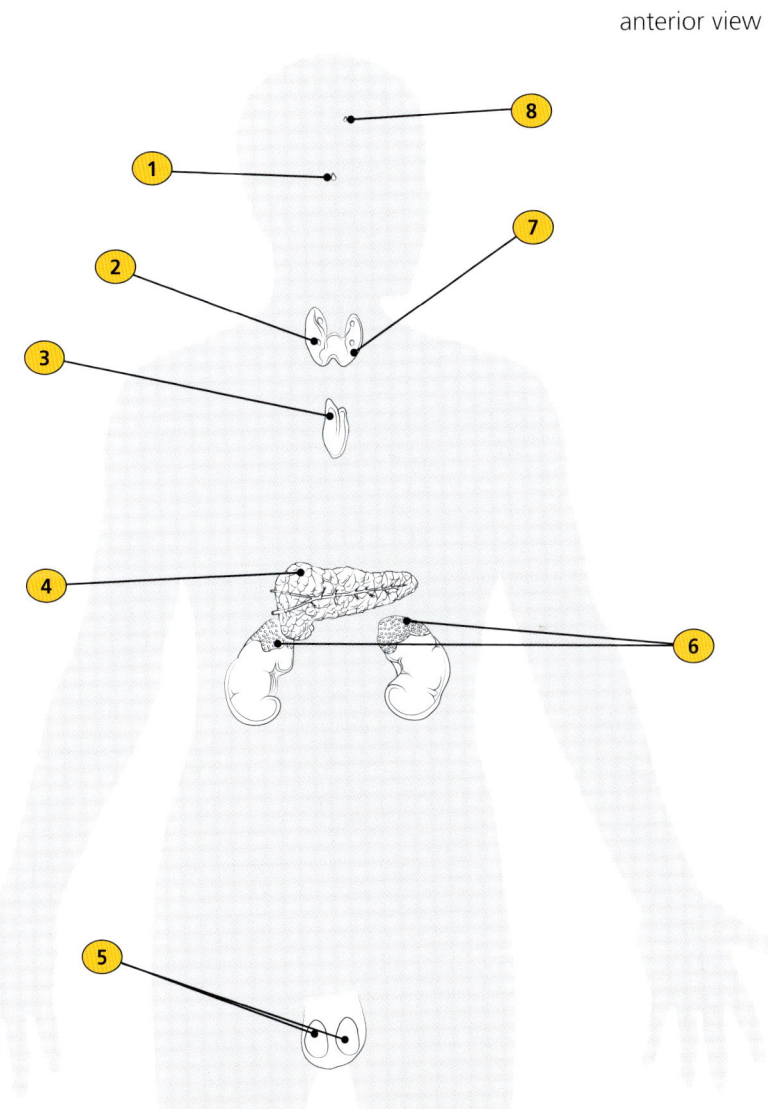

Endocrine System: Female

Key:

1 Pituitary gland
2 Parathyroid gland (on back of thyroid gland lobe)
3 Thymus gland (atrophic in adults)
4 Pancreas
5 Ovaries
6 Adrenal glands (includes cortex and medulla)
7 Thyroid gland
8 Pineal gland

Description:

The endocrine organs (or endocrine glands) secrete hormones that regulate growth, metabolism, sexual maturation, and other important body functions.

The organs involved in the female endocrine system include the pituitary, pineal, thymus, thyroid, parathyroids, adrenals, pancreatic islets, ovaries, and placenta (during pregnancy). The ovaries produce hormones that control sexual function and secondary sexual characteristics.

anterior view

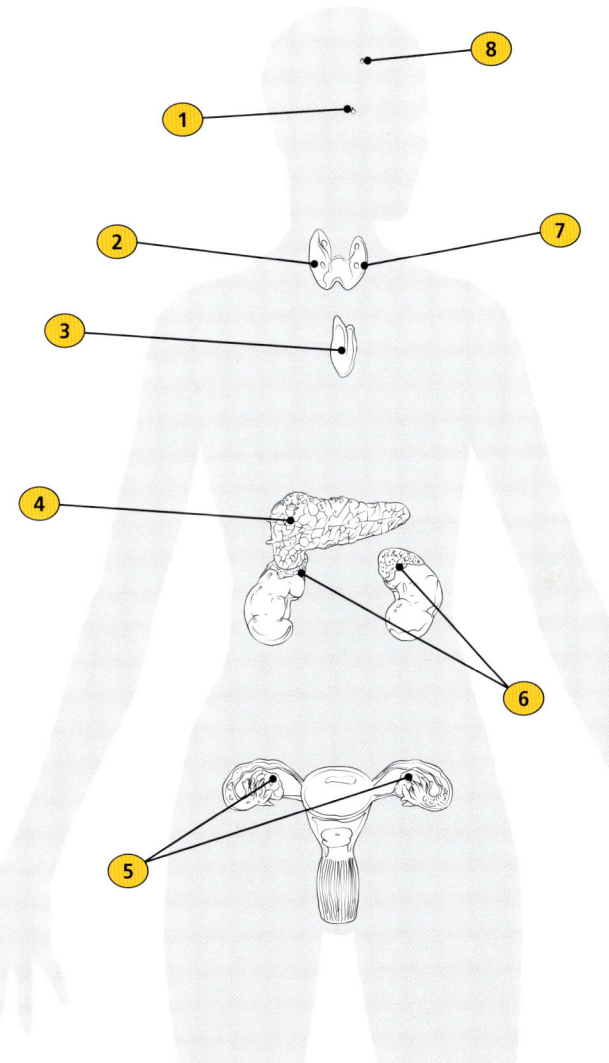

Pituitary Gland

Key:

1 Optic chiasm
2 Infundibulum
3 Hypophyseal artery
4 Anterior pituitary (adenohypophysis)
5 Posterior pituitary (neurohypophysis)
6 Hypophyseal portal system
7 Parvocellular neurosecretory axon
8 Mammillary body
9 Hypothalamus
10 Magnocellular neurosecretory cells

Description:
The pituitary gland (hypophysis) is a very small organ lying immediately below the hypothalamus of the brain. It plays a very important role in the control of endocrine gland function throughout the body.

The pituitary gland is divided into anterior and posterior lobes—the adenohypophysis and neurohypophysis, respectively. The anterior lobe contains many different types of cells, which produce growth hormone, prolactin, follicle-stimulating hormone, luteinizing hormone, thyroid-stimulating hormone, adrenocorticotrophic hormone, and melanocyte-stimulating hormone. The production of hormones by the anterior pituitary is controlled by regulatory factors released from parvocellular neurosecretory axons into the hypophyseal portal system. These regulatory factors are carried to the anterior pituitary by the blood flow of the portal system.

The posterior lobe contains oxytocin and antidiuretic hormones, produced in the hypothalamus and transported to the pituitary in nerve fibers of magnocellular neurosecretory cells.

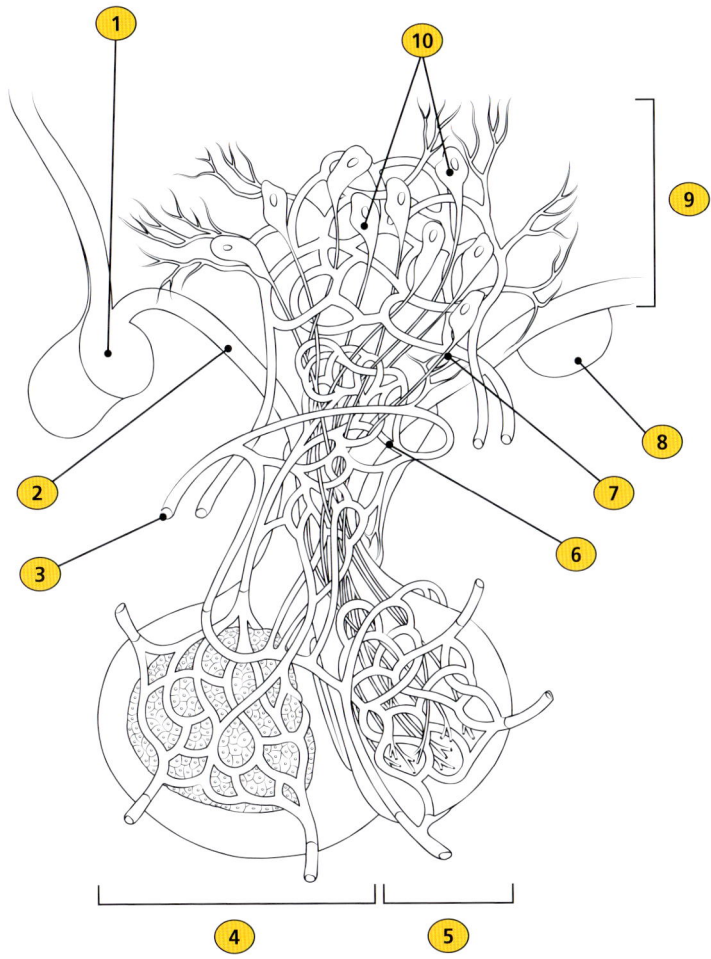

Pineal Gland

Key:

1 Pineal gland
2 Brainstem
3 Cerebellum
4 Cerebrum (medial surface)

Description:

The small pineal gland (body) is located inside the skull cavity, surrounded by the brain. It produces melatonin, whose concentration varies in tune with the 24-hour cycle of the day (circadian rhythm)—melatonin production is highest during a person's normal sleeping hours and drops off as the body begins to wake. The pineal gland probably has an effect on the ovaries and testes, and may influence mood. In older people, the pineal gland may calcify and appear on skull X-rays and computed tomography, or CT, scans.

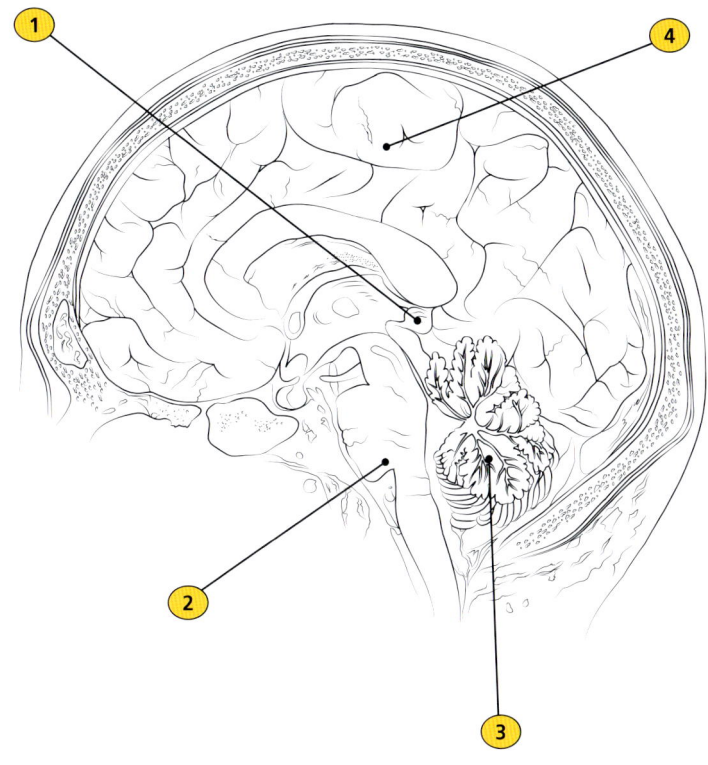

Thyroid Gland

Key:

1 Thyroid cartilage (of larynx)
2 Cricoid cartilage (of larynx)
3 Right lobe of thyroid gland
4 Trachea
5 Isthmus of thyroid gland
6 Left lobe of thyroid gland

Description:

The largest of the endocrine glands, the thyroid gland, consists of two lobes, joined together at the midline by a narrow isthmus (bridge). The thyroid gland is located in the neck, immediately below, and in front of, the larynx.

The thyroid gland is made up of many follicles that produce thyroid hormone and secrete it into the bloodstream. Thyroid hormone is composed of two different substances—thyroxine (also called T4, or tetraiodothyronine) and tri-iodothyronine (T3). Thyroid hormone has several functions, the main one being to control the metabolic rate of body tissues. The production of thyroid hormone is under the control of thyroid-stimulating hormone (TSH), which is released from the anterior pituitary gland. Thyroid hormone is necessary for the normal growth and development of children and normal brain development.

The thyroid gland also contains parafollicular cells that produce thyrocalcitonin (or calcitonin), which controls calcium metabolism.

anterior view

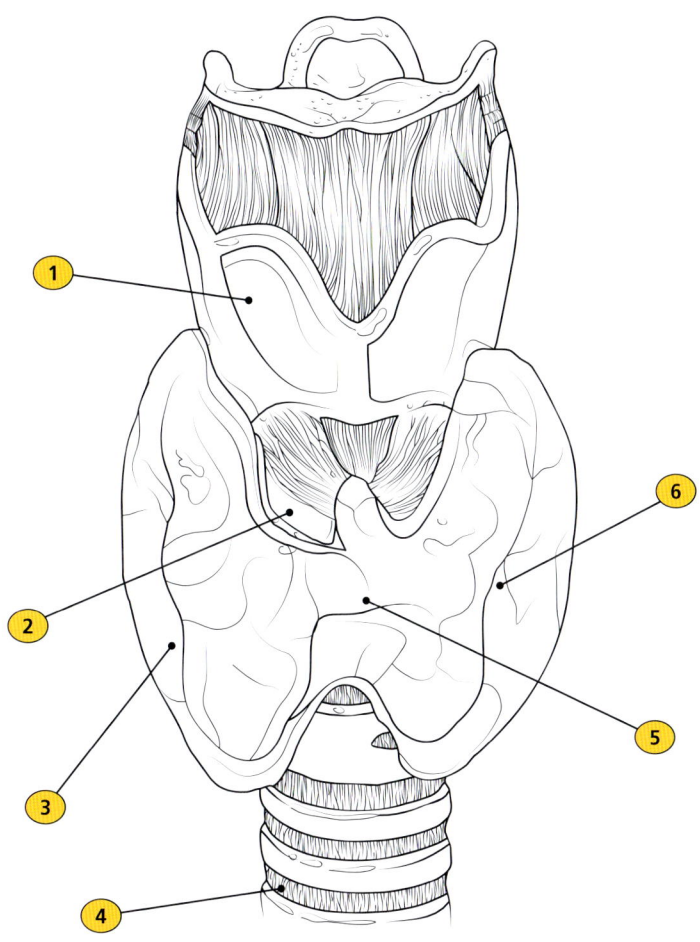

Parathyroid Glands

Key:

1 Pharyngeal muscles (superior, middle, and inferior constrictors)
2 Thyroid gland
3 Esophagus
4 Parathyroid glands

Description:

The parathyroid glands are four (or occasionally three) pea-sized endocrine glands, which lie just behind the thyroid gland in the neck. Each parathyroid gland has a fibrous tissue capsule and two types of cells—chief cells and oxyphil cells. Chief cells produce parathyroid hormone, which acts to raise the concentration of calcium in the blood and reduce the concentration of phosphate ions. The role of oxyphil cells is unclear, although they may be transitional chief cells.

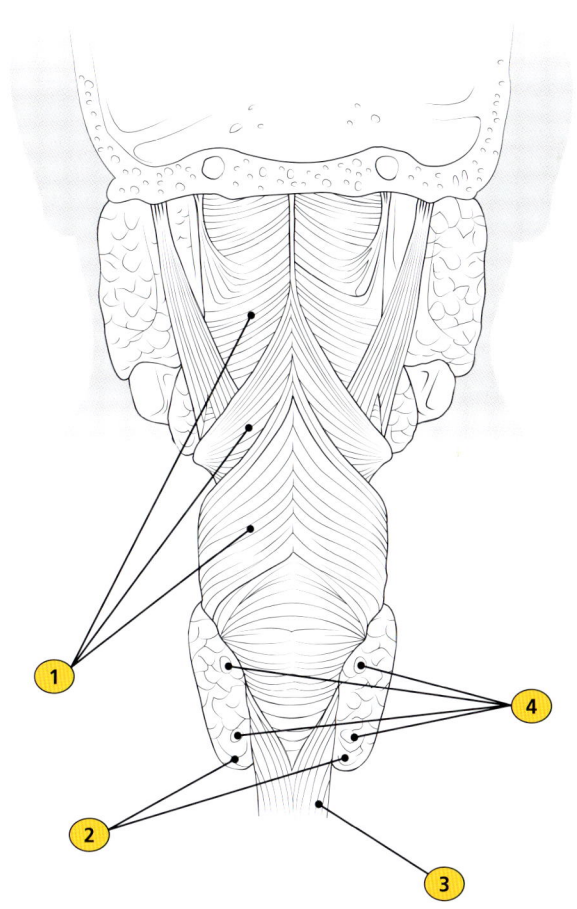

Thyroid and Parathyroid Glands

Key:

1 Lumen filled with colloid
2 Thyroid epithelium   } Thyroid Follicle
3 Capsule of parathyroid
4 Chief cell
5 Capillary   } Parathyroid
6 Oxyphil cells

Description:

The thyroid gland consists of two lobes joined together at the midline. The thyroid gland is located in the neck, immediately below, and in front of, the larynx, and is made up of many follicles. These make thyroid hormones, which have as their main function control of the metabolic rate of body tissues. Each follicle consists of thyroid epithelial cells arranged around a cavity (or lumen) filled with colloid, a gelatinous substance. Thyroid hormones are stored within the colloid.

The parathyroid glands are four (or occasionally three) pea-sized endocrine glands, which lie just behind the thyroid gland. Each parathyroid gland has a fibrous tissue capsule and two types of cells—chief cells and oxyphil cells. Chief cells produce parathyroid hormone when calcium levels in the blood fall.

microstructure

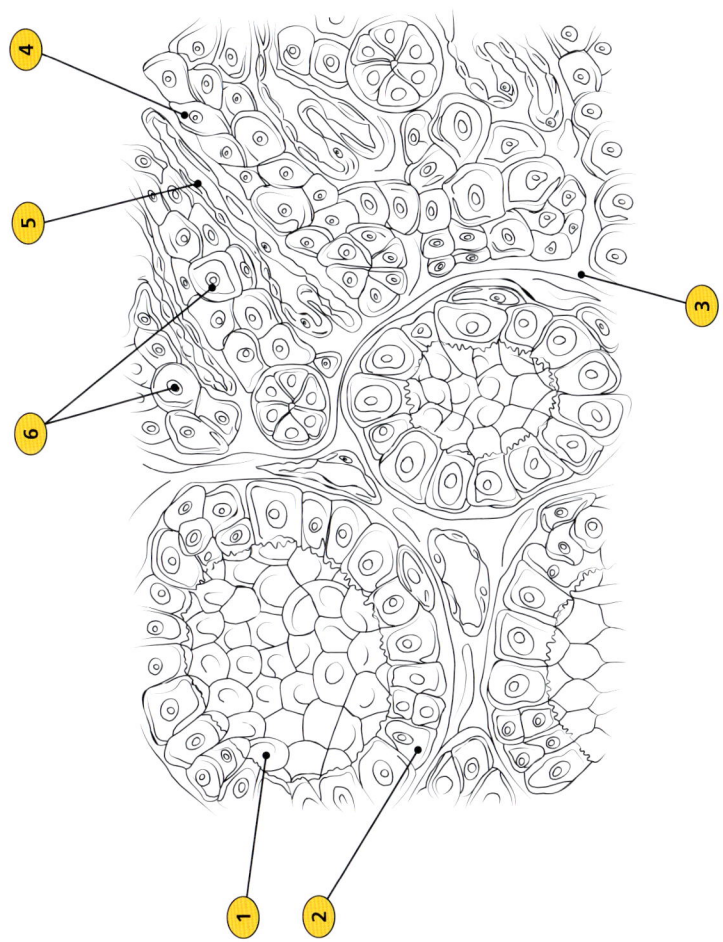

Endocrine System

Islets of Langerhans

Key:

1 Islet of Langerhans
2 Exocrine pancreas
3 Insuloacinar portal vessels

Description:
The pancreas is an elongated gland lying behind the stomach. The pancreas plays a role in both the digestive and endocrine systems. Its endocrine function is hormonal and is involved in regulation of glucose mobilization and storage (the responsible hormones are glucagon and insulin, respectively). These two hormones are produced in special cell types (alpha and beta cells, respectively) within many tiny spherical clumps of pancreatic tissue, known as pancreatic islets or the islets of Langerhans. The islets are surrounded by exocrine tissue that produces digestive enzymes, which are secreted into the second part of the duodenum.

microstructure

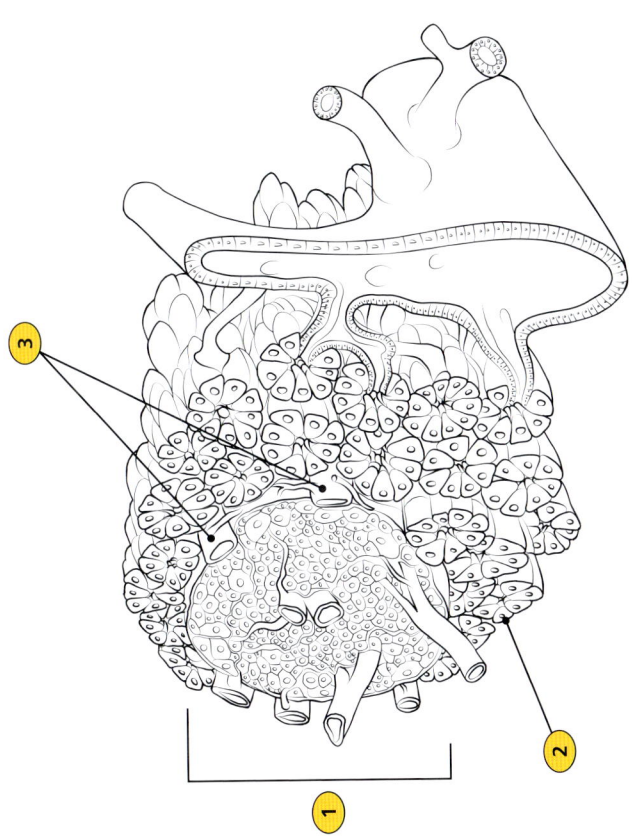

Adrenal Glands

Key:
1 Left suprarenal artery
2 Left adrenal medulla
3 Left kidney capsule
4 Left adrenal gland
5 Left adrenal cortex

Description:

The two adrenal (or suprarenal) glands lie one on top of each kidney at the back of the abdomen. Each adrenal gland is 1–2 inches (3–5 cm) long, somewhat triangular in shape, and yellowish brown in color. Each gland has an outer part (the cortex) and a core (the medulla).

The adrenal cortex produces three main types of hormones—glucocorticoids, mineralocorticoids, and sex steroids. Glucocorticoids, produced and released under the control of adrenocorticotrophic hormone (ACTH) from the anterior pituitary, influence the metabolism of fat, protein, and carbohydrates, promoting the breakdown of protein and the release of fat and sugars into the bloodstream. Mineralocorticoids regulate the release of sodium in the kidneys. Sex steroids contribute to the development of sexual characteristics and libido.

The adrenal medulla contains many modified nerve cells, which produce the hormones epinephrine and norepinephrine (adrenaline and noradrenaline, respectively). These hormones are released in bursts during emergency situations or accompanying intense emotion. They act to increase the strength and rate of heart contraction, raise the blood sugar level, and elevate blood pressure.

coronal section through left adrenal gland

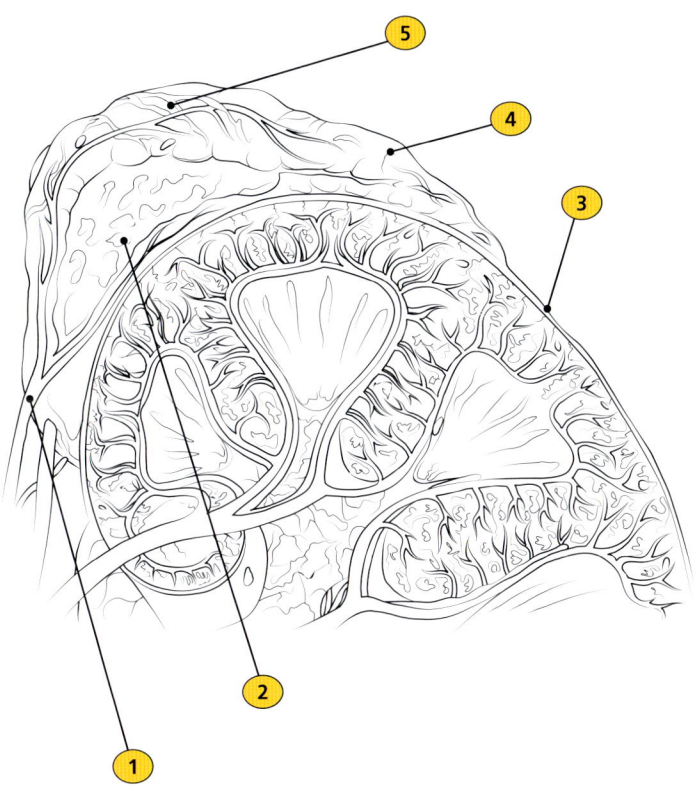

Endocrine System

Adrenal Gland

Key:

1 Zona glomerulosa
2 Zona fasciculata
3 Zona reticularis
4 Medullary plexus of veins
5 Medullary vein
6 Medulla

7 Deep plexus of veins
8 Sinusoidal vessels
9 Subcapsular plexus of veins
10 Capsular artery
11 Capsule

Description:

The two triangular adrenal (or suprarenal) glands lie one on top of each kidney at the back of the abdomen. Each gland has an outer part (the cortex) and a core (the medulla). The adrenal cortex produces three main types of hormones—glucocorticoids, mineralocorticoids, and sex steroids. Glucocorticoids promote the breakdown of protein and the release of fat and sugars into the bloodstream. Mineralocorticoids regulate the release of sodium in the kidneys. Sex steroids contribute to the development of sexual characteristics and libido.

The adrenal medulla contains many modified nerve cells, which produce the hormones epinephrine and norepinephrine (adrenaline and noradrenaline, respectively). These hormones are released in bursts during emergency situations or accompanying intense emotion. They act to increase the strength and rate of heart contraction, raise the blood sugar level, elevate blood pressure, and dilate the airways.

microstructure

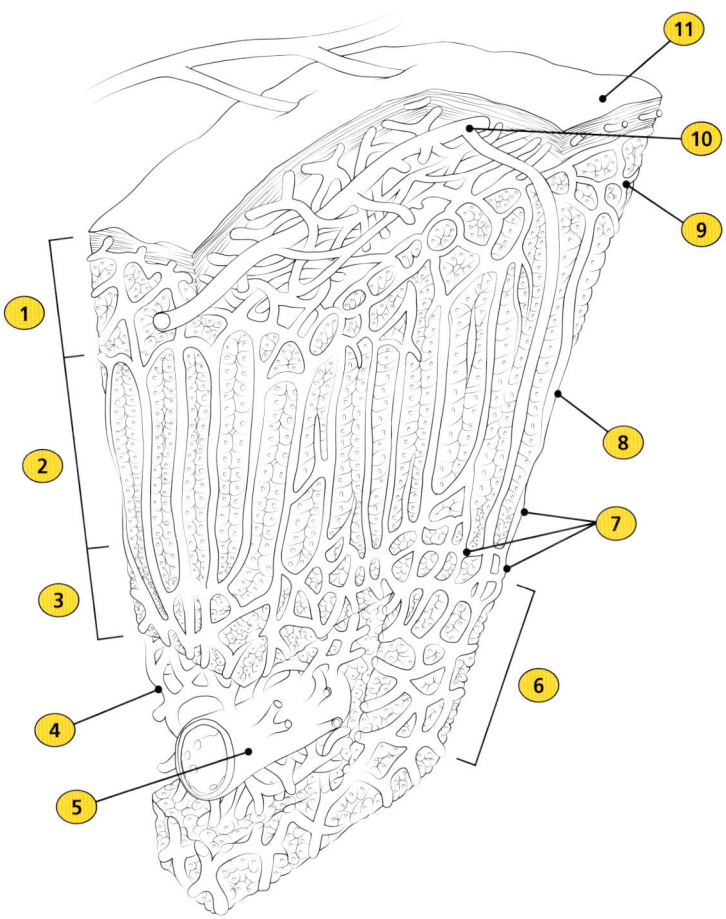

Endocrine System

Endocrine Cells in the Testes

Key:

1 Spermatocytes
2 Sertoli cells
3 Spermatids
4 Seminiferous tubule
5 Interstitial cell (Leydig cell)
6 Spermatozoa
7 Spermatogonia

Description:

The testes are two ovoid organs contained in the scrotum. The testes function as endocrine glands, producing hormones that control sexual function and secondary sexual characteristics (primarily testosterone).

The testes are separated by a central partition. Surrounding each testis is a double-layered membrane, the tunica vaginalis. Each testis has a tough inelastic fibrous wall called the tunica albuginea, which sends partitions inward to divide it into about 300 lobules. Each lobule contains coiled seminiferous tubules that produce sperm, and converge into a network that sends about 20 small ducts through the tunica albuginea into the epididymis.

The germ cells in the seminiferous tubules, the spermatogonia, undergo division (meiosis) to become spermatids. Spermatids mature into sperm that have a head and a long tail. The head is capped by an acrosome, which releases enzymes to help the sperm penetrate the ovum (egg). The spaces between the seminiferous tubules contain clumps of endocrine cells called interstitial cells (or Leydig cells). These interstitial cells synthesize the male hormone testosterone, responsible for the development of sexual characteristics in the adolesent male and the functioning of the reproductive system.

microstructure

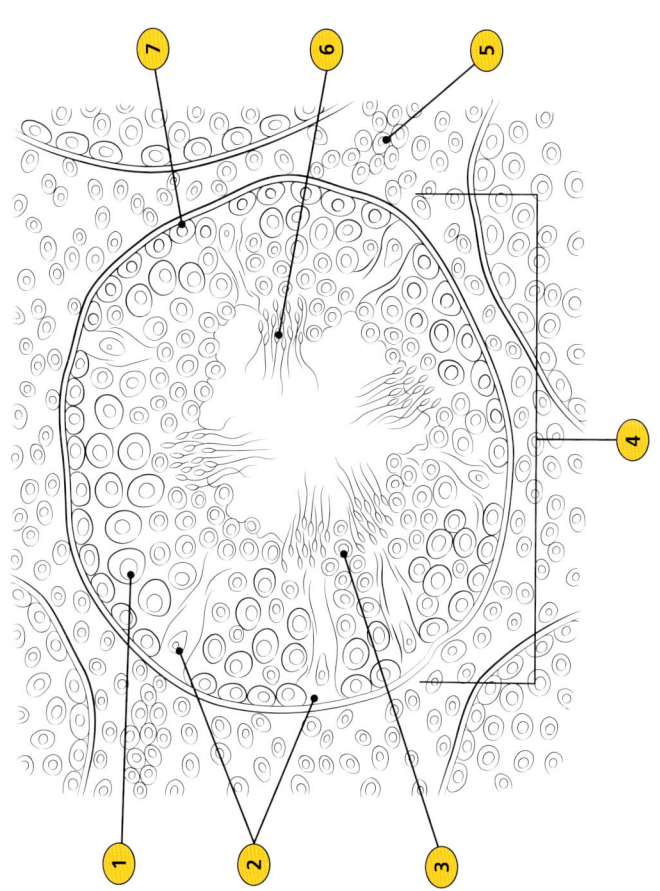

Ovaries

Key:
1 Uterine tube
2 Mature ovum
3 Discharging follicle (at ovulation)
4 Ovum
5 Ovary
6 Uterus
7 Vagina
8 Corpus albicans
9 Corpus luteum

Description:
The two ovaries are the female gonads in which the ova are formed. They resemble almonds in shape and are situated on either side of the uterus, supported by the broad ligament. The ovaries produce the female hormones estrogen and progesterone. Estrogen causes growth of the breasts and reproductive organs, among other functions. Progesterone maintains the lining of the uterus in a state suitable to receive and nourish a fertilized ovum.

Estrogen and progesterone undergo cyclical changes in level every 28 days under the influence of follicle-stimulating hormone (FSH) and luteinizing hormone (LH), which are secreted by the anterior lobe of the pituitary gland. The corpus luteum is produced after release of the ovum and, if fertilization occurs, produces estrogen and progesterone to maintain the early embryo.

posterosuperior view

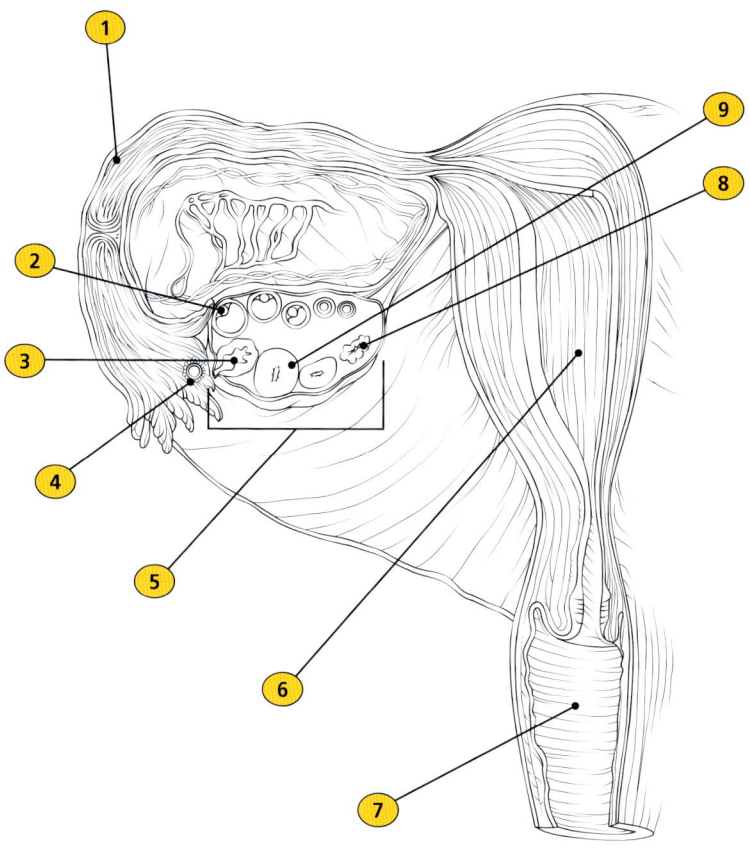

Placenta

Key:

1 Amnion
2 Branch of umbilical vein
3 Branch of umbilical artery
4 Cotyledon (on maternal side)
5 Umbilical cord

Description:

An organ of pregnancy, the placenta connects the baby to the mother via the umbilical cord. It ensures that the baby receives adequate nutrients and oxygen.

The placenta also acts as an endocrine organ, producing a hormone to sustain the pregnancy (human chorionic gonadotrophin, or HCG). HCG is the earliest placental hormone to be produced and is first secreted on day six of gestation. HCG maintains the corpus luteum (the ovarian follicle from which the ovum burst) and ensures that it continues to manufacture progesterone and estrogen until the placenta is able to produce adequate amounts of both, usually by the third month of gestation, when HCG levels decline. The placenta also produces estrogen, progesterone, and relaxin (which relaxes the pelvic ligaments), along with human placental lactogen, which promotes milk production and fetal growth.

amniotic surface and umbilical cord

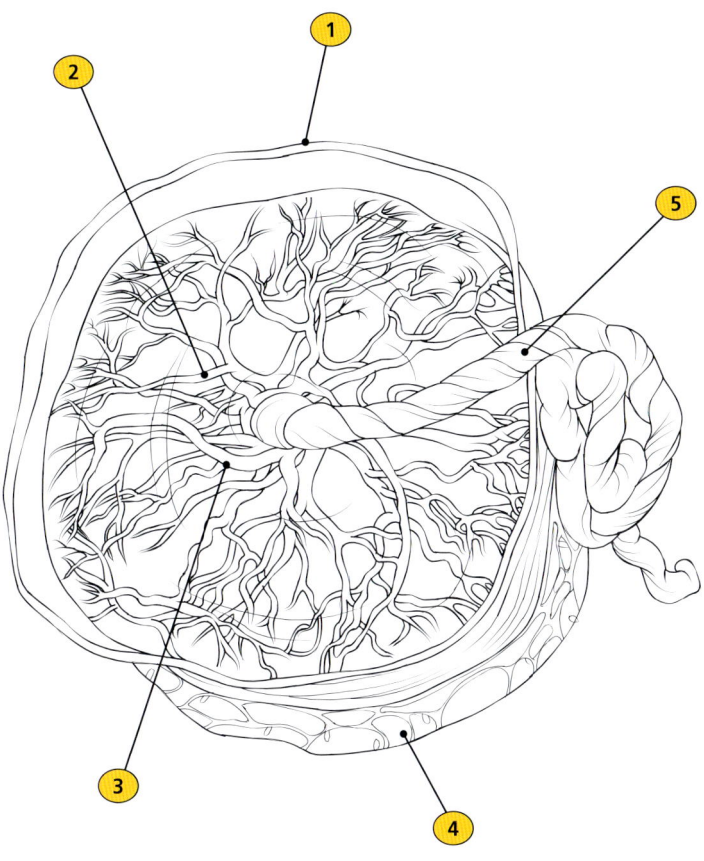

Placenta

Key:

1 Area filled with maternal blood
2 Placenta
3 Endometrium
4 Myometrium
5 Maternal blood vessels
6 Chorionic villi
7 Syncytial trophoblast
8 Umbilical arteries
9 Umbilical vein
10 Umbilical cord

Description:

The placenta contains tissue from both the mother and baby, allowing for the diffusion of nutrients and oxygen, and the removal of fetal waste. The placenta forms a protective barrier between the maternal and fetal blood. The placenta also acts as an endocrine organ, producing a hormone to sustain the pregnancy (human chorionic gonadotrophin, or HCG). The placenta also produces estrogen, progesterone, and relaxin (which relaxes the pelvic ligaments in preparation for parturition, or delivery of the baby), along with human placental lactogen, which promotes milk production and fetal growth.

cross-sectional view

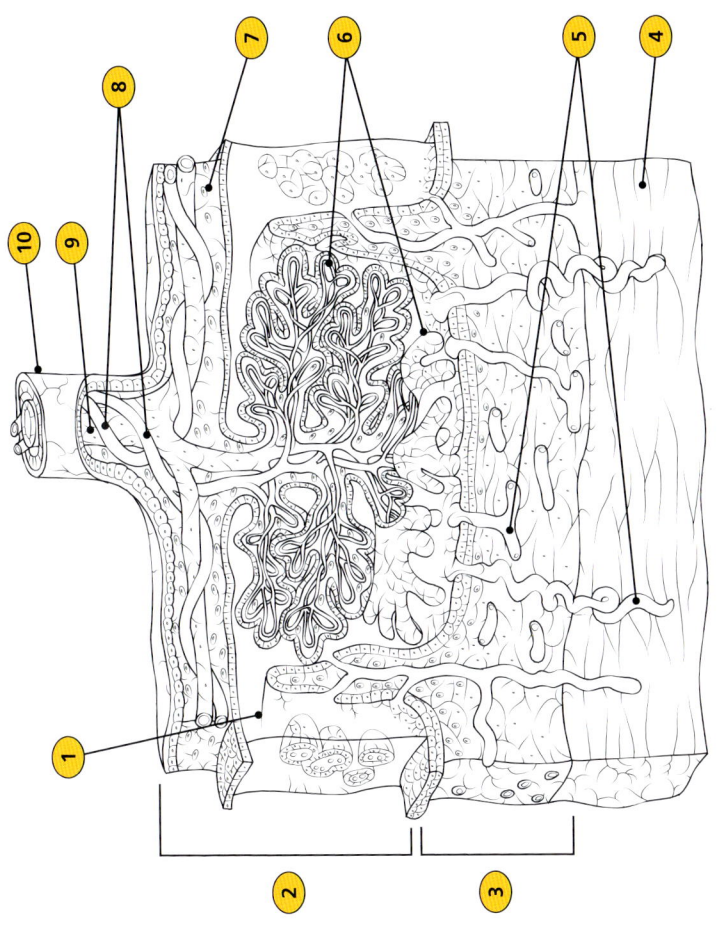

Circulatory System

The role of the circulatory system is to move blood and its constituent cells and chemicals around the body. This requires a pump (the heart) plus a complex network of vessels. The circulatory system is divided into two circulations: a pulmonary circulation solely for gas exchange in the lungs; and a systemic circulation to carry oxygenated and nutrient-rich blood to the other organs, and to return waste and carbon dioxide back to the heart. The systemic and pulmonary circulations both consist of high-pressure vessels (arteries); microvasculature beds for exchange of gases, nutrients, and waste (capillaries); and a reservoir compartment (veins).

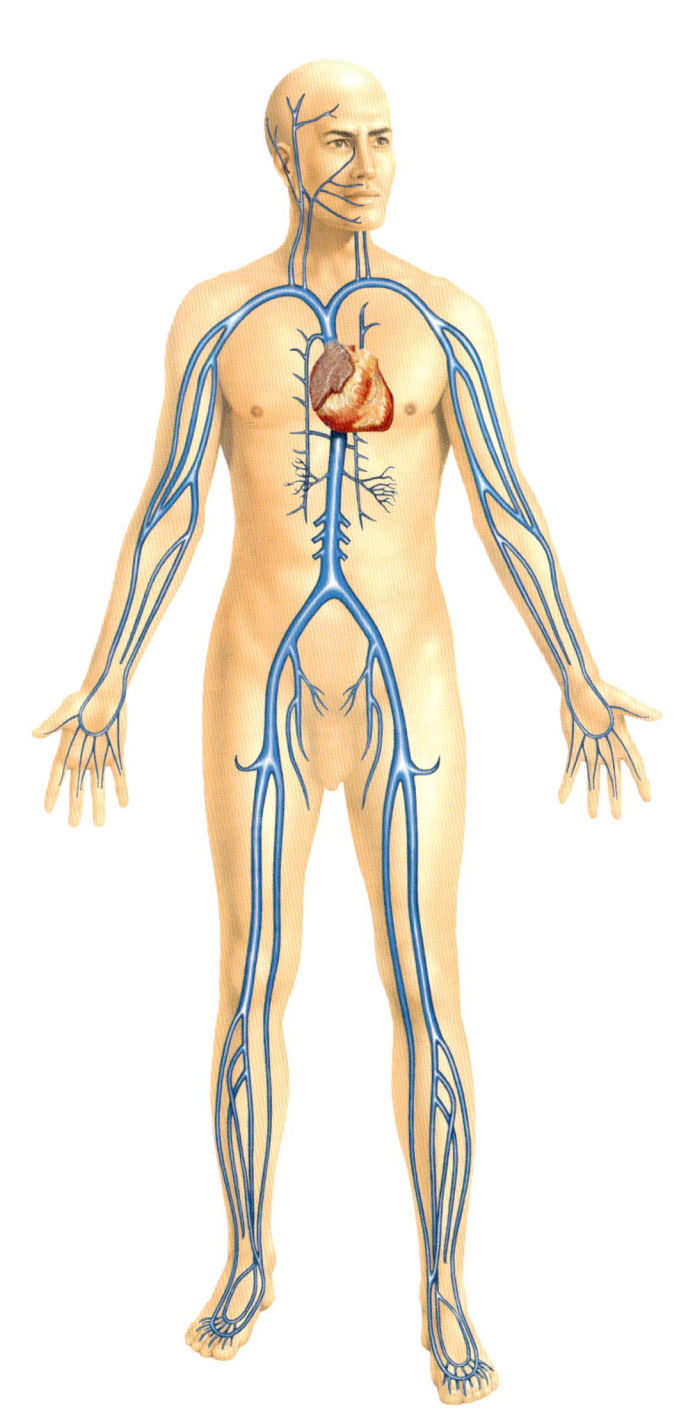

Circulatory System

Key:

1 Common carotid artery
2 External jugular vein
3 Axillary vein
4 Superior vena cava
5 Brachial artery
6 Common iliac vein
7 Radial vein
8 Ulnar artery
9 Common iliac artery
10 Basilic vein
11 Inferior vena cava
12 Cephalic vein
13 Heart
14 Thoracic descending aorta
15 Left subclavian vein

Description:

The circulatory system includes the heart and blood vessels, which form a closed circuit. The heart has four chambers. It propels blood out from its two major pumps—the left and right ventricles—and collects returned blood into its left and right atria. Blood is pumped out of the left and right ventricles through arteries into a distribution network of capillaries. After exchanging gases and nutrients with surrounding tissues, blood returns to the left and right atria, respectively, via the veins.

There are two separate parts (or circuits) in the circulatory system, which are connected through the heart. In the systemic circulation, blood from the left ventricle of the heart is distributed throughout the body to deliver oxygen and nutrients to the entire body, and returns to the right atrium.

Continued on page 44

anterior view

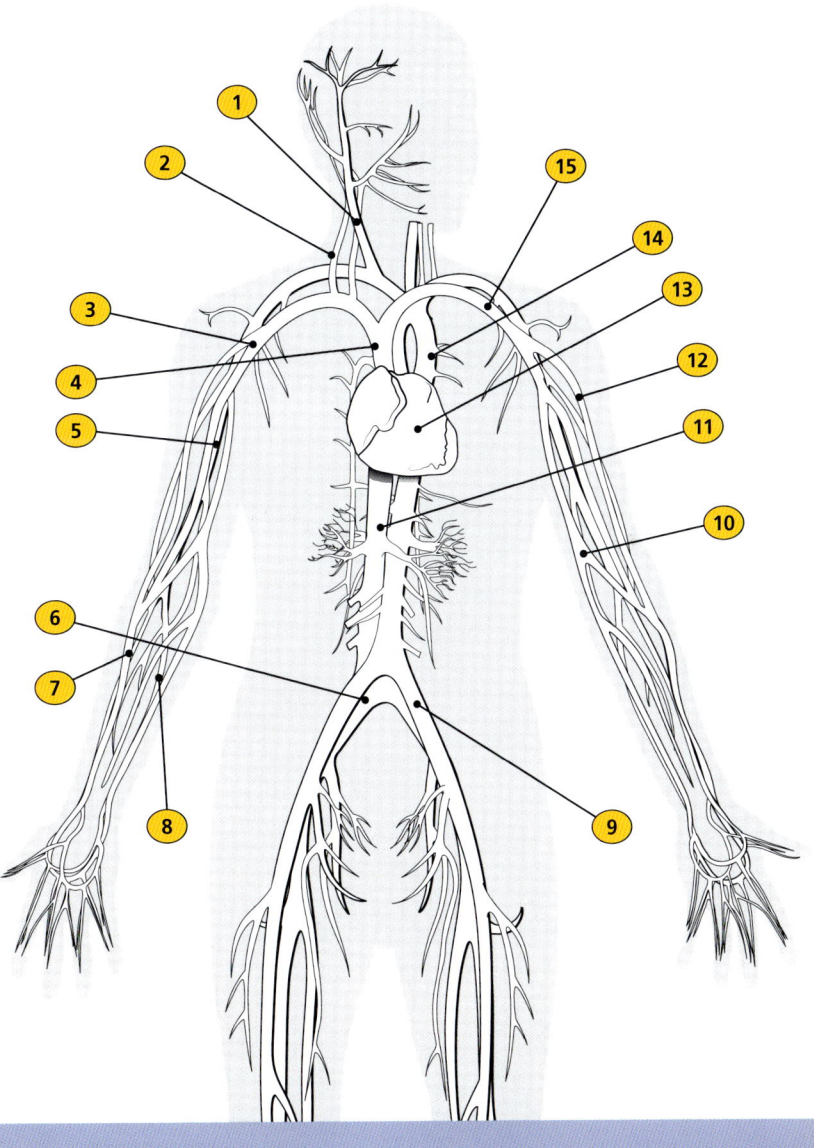

Circulatory System

Key:

1 Femoral artery
2 Anterior tibial artery
3 Posterior tibial artery
4 Great saphenous vein
5 Fibular artery
6 Small saphenous vein
7 Popliteal vein
8 Obturator artery
9 Obturator vein

Description:

Continued from page 42

Blood returning to the right atrium is depleted of oxygen and loaded with carbon dioxide. This blood then flows into the right ventricle, where it is pumped into the capillary network in the lungs (pulmonary circulation), from where, after exchanging carbon dioxide for oxygen, blood is returned to the left atrium. From the left atrium, blood flows to the left ventricle, and the cycle continues.

The major arteries of the systemic circulation are derived from the aorta—these are the carotid arteries for the head and neck, the axillary arteries for the upper limbs, and the iliac arteries for the pelvis and lower limbs. There are two main systemic veins—the superior vena cava, which returns blood from the head and upper limbs, and the inferior vena cava, which returns blood from the lower limbs and abdomen. The four pulmonary veins return oxygenated blood to the left atrium.

Note: The small saphenous vein has been deliberately displaced laterally for illustrative reasons and usually runs up the posterior surface of the calf.

anterior view

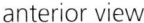

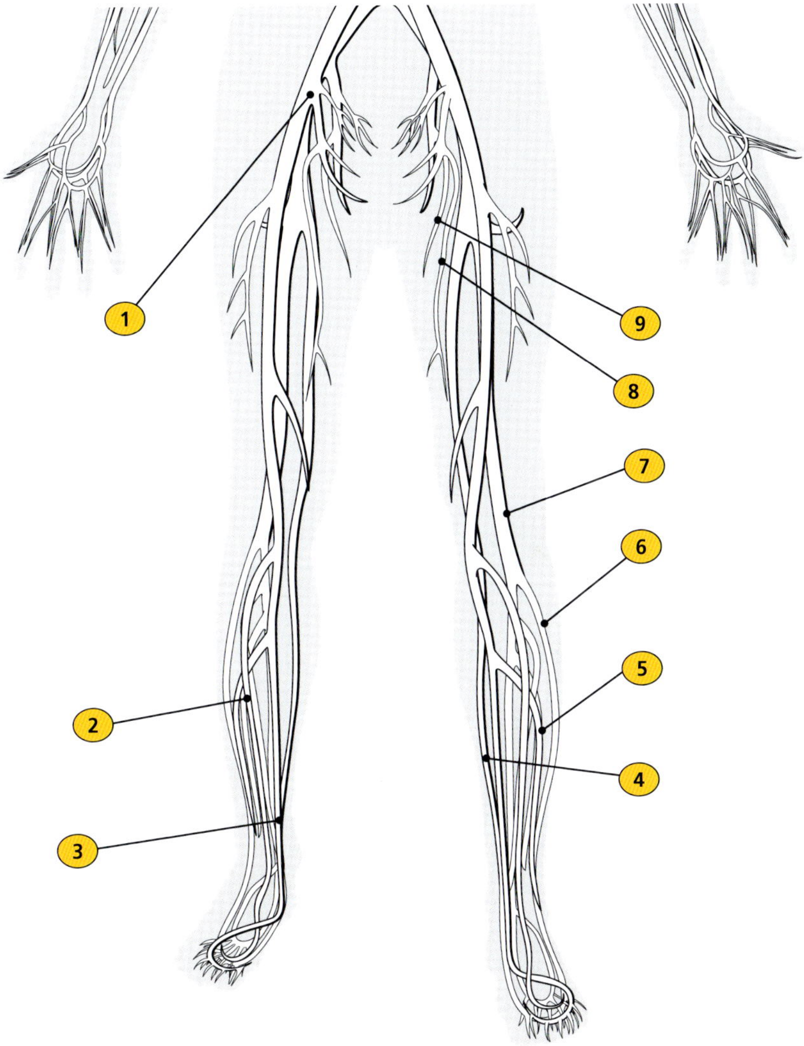

1

2

3

4

5

6

7

8

9

Circulatory System

Heart

Key:

1 Brachiocephalic artery
2 Right brachiocephalic vein
3 Superior vena cava
4 Right atrium
5 Right pulmonary artery
6 Right superior pulmonary vein
7 Right inferior pulmonary vein
8 Right coronary artery
9 Right ventricle
10 Inferior vena cava
11 Descending thoracic aorta
12 Left ventricle
13 Anterior descending branch of left coronary artery
14 Left atrium
15 Left inferior pulmonary vein
16 Left superior pulmonary vein
17 Left pulmonary artery
18 Aortic arch
19 Left brachiocephalic vein
20 Left subclavian artery
21 Left common carotid artery

Description:

The heart lies in the midline of the thorax (mediastinum), between the lungs, surrounded by the double-layered membrane of the pericardium. The right and left atria are located at the back, and the right and left ventricles at the front. The interatrial septum divides the right and left atria, and the interventricular septum separates the right and left ventricles. Each atrium opens into the respective ventricle through an atrioventricular orifice, which is guarded by a valve to ensure that blood flows in only one direction.

anterior view

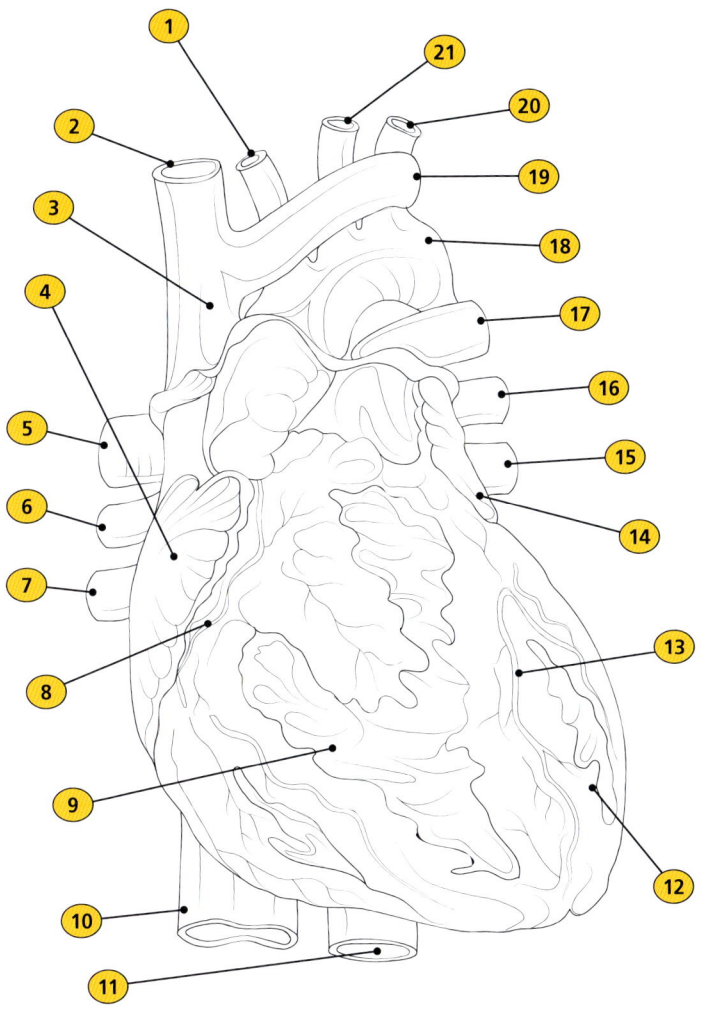

Circulatory System

Heart

Key:

1 Left subclavian artery
2 Aortic arch
3 Left pulmonary artery
4 Pericardium
5 Right pulmonary artery
6 Left superior pulmonary vein
7 Left inferior pulmonary vein
8 Left ventricle
9 Right ventricle

10 Right coronary artery
11 Inferior vena cava
12 Right atrium
13 Right inferior pulmonary vein
14 Right superior pulmonary vein
15 Superior vena cava
16 Brachiocephalic artery
17 Left common carotid artery

Description:

The heart lies in the midline of the thorax (mediastinum), between the lungs, surrounded by the double-layered membrane of the pericardium. The right and left atria are located at the back, and the right and left ventricles at the front. The interatrial septum divides the right and left atria, and the interventricular septum separates the right and left ventricles. Each atrium opens into the respective ventricle through an atrioventricular orifice, which is guarded by a valve to ensure that blood flows in only one direction.

posterior view

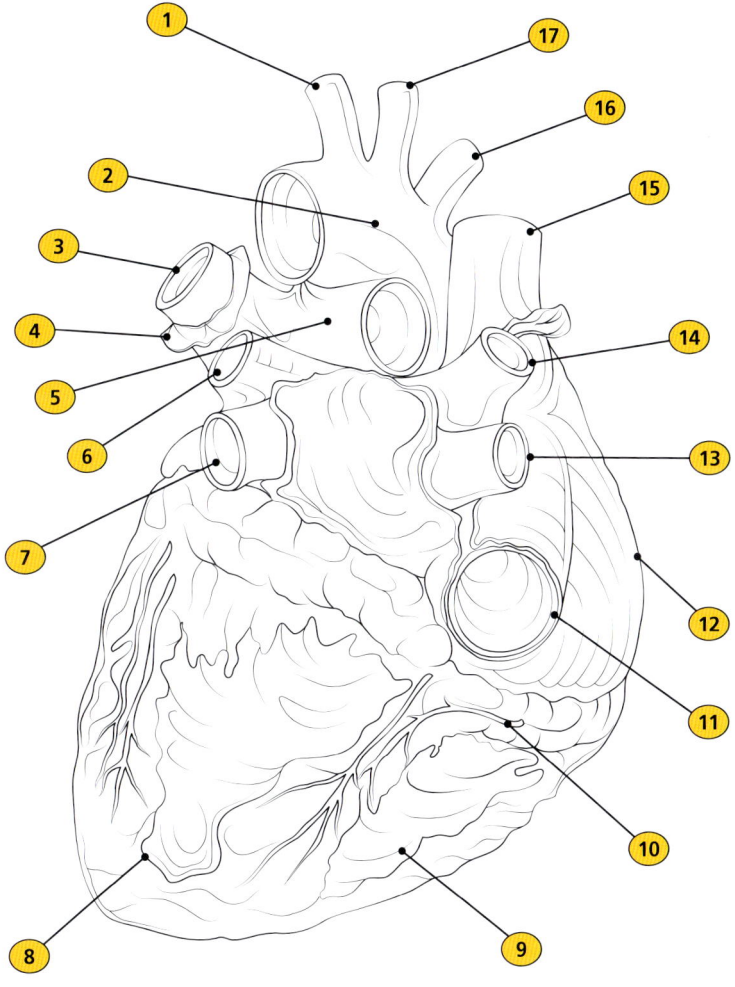

Circulatory System

Heart

Key:

1 Brachiocephalic artery
2 Right brachiocephalic vein
3 Superior vena cava
4 Ascending aorta
5 Right pulmonary artery
6 Right superior pulmonary vein
7 Right inferior pulmonary vein
8 Pulmonary valve
9 Right atrium
10 Cusp of tricuspid valve
11 Right ventricle
12 Papillary muscles
13 Inferior vena cava
14 Descending thoracic aorta
15 Chordae tendineae
16 Cusp of mitral valve
17 Cusp of aortic valve
18 Left atrium
19 Left inferior pulmonary vein
20 Left superior pulmonary vein
21 Pericardium
22 Left pulmonary artery
23 Ligamentum arteriosum
24 Aortic arch
25 Left brachiocephalic vein
26 Left subclavian artery
27 Left common carotid artery

Description:

A cross-sectional view of the heart exposes the four chambers and valves. On the left side of the heart are the left atrium and ventricle, between which the mitral valve sits. Blood exiting from the left ventricle is released through the aortic valve. On the right side of the heart are the right atrium and ventricle, between which the tricuspid valve sits. Blood leaving the right ventricle passes through the pulmonary valve.

cross-sectional view

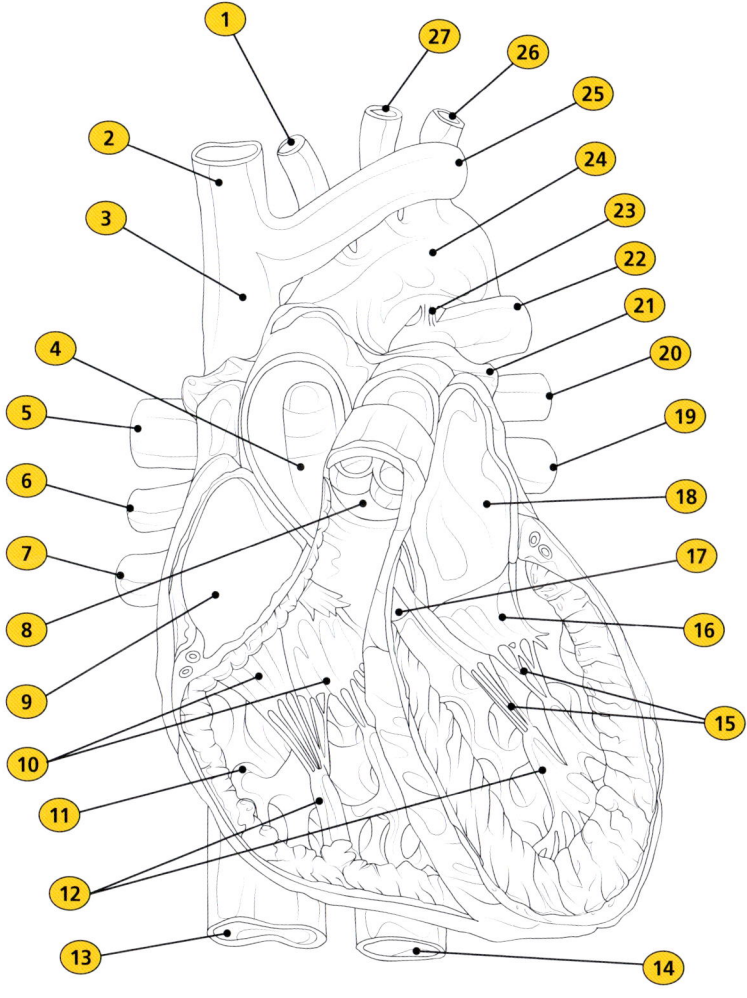

Heart Valves: Ventricular Systole

Key:

1 Pulmonary valve (open)

2 Mitral valve

3 Tricuspid valve

4 Aortic valve (open)

Description:

The four valves of the heart are designed to allow one-way flow of blood. Their function is to prevent backflow into the releasing chamber. The atrioventricular valves—the mitral and tricuspid valves—separate the atrium and ventricle on the left and right sides of the heart, respectively. During ventricular systole, the ventricles of the heart contract and the pulmonary and aortic valves open to allow blood to be pumped into the pulmonary and systemic circulatory systems, respectively, while the mitral and tricuspid valves remain closed.

The aortic and pulmonary valves are said to be semilunar valves, because each consists of three half-moon-shaped valve cusps that are attached to the inside wall of the aortic and pulmonary arteries.

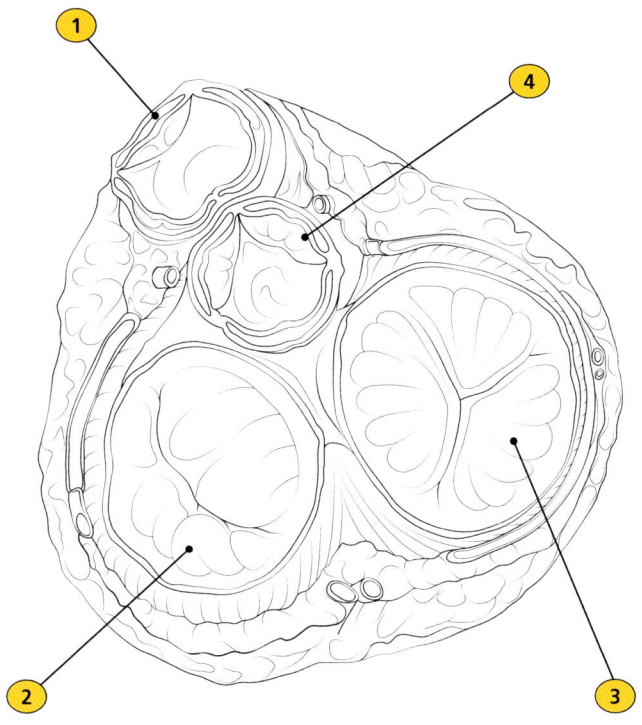

Circulatory System

Heart Valves: Ventricular Diastole

Key:

1 Pulmonary valve
2 Papillary muscles
3 Mitral valve (open)
4 Chordae tendineae
5 Tricuspid valve (open)
6 Aortic valve

Description:

The four heart valves work in pairs in tandem. During ventricular diastole, the aortic and pulmonary valves close, while the atrioventricular valves—the tricuspid and mitral valves—open to allow blood to pass from the atria to the ventricles.

The cusps of the atrioventricular valves have the tough fibrous cords of the chordae tendineae attached along their free edge. The other ends of the chordae tendineae are attached to the papillary muscles, which are designed to pull down on the chordae and valve cusps when the ventricle contracts, thus keeping the valves shut, as the ventricles rapidly decrease in size during contraction.

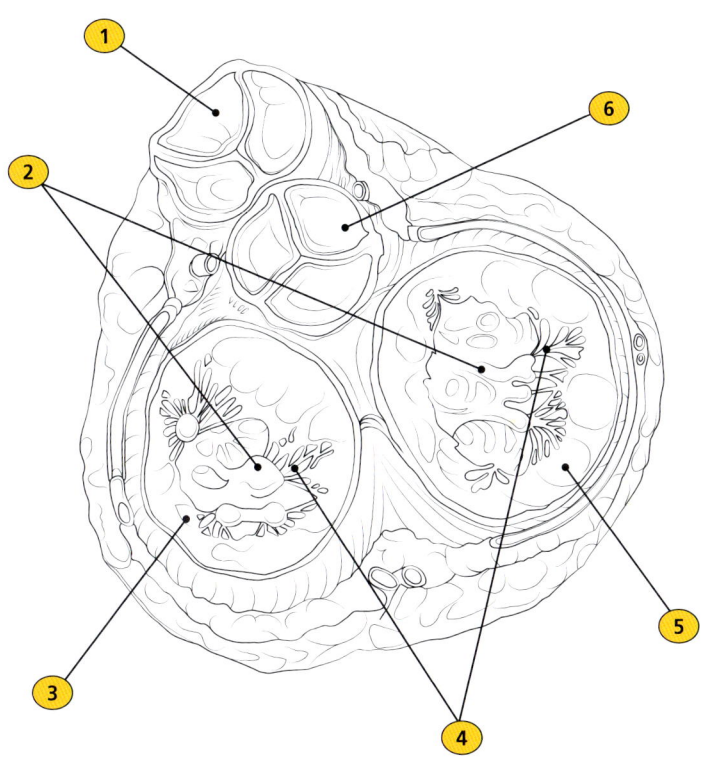

Major Arteries of the Circulatory System

Key:

1	Common carotid artery	**8**	Palmar arches
2	Heart	**9**	Ulnar artery
3	Brachial artery	**10**	Radial artery
4	Renal artery	**11**	Abdominal aorta
5	Common iliac artery	**12**	Arch of aorta
6	External iliac artery	**13**	Axillary artery
7	Internal iliac artery	**14**	Facial artery

Description:

The largest artery is the aorta, which channels blood from the heart to other arteries, and then to the body's organs and other structures.
Two small branches of the aorta, the coronary arteries, supply blood to the heart muscle itself. The right and left carotid arteries carry blood to the two sides of the neck and head. Blood flows to the shoulders and upper limbs through the right and left subclavian arteries. In the abdomen, the aorta divides into two large branches, the left and right common iliacs, supplying blood to the pelvic region and lower limbs. The external iliac arteries then continue into the lower limbs, where they become the femoral arteries.

Continued on page 58

anterior view

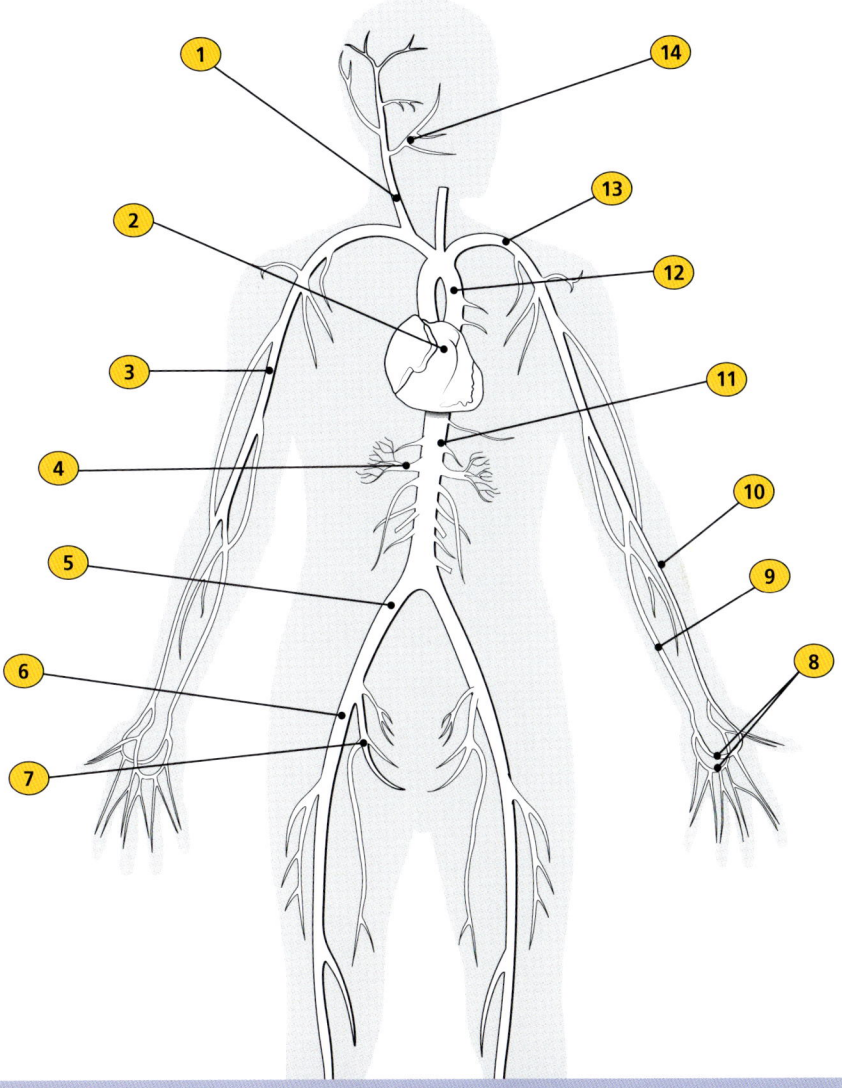

Circulatory System

Major Arteries of the Circulatory System

Key:

1 Obturator artery
2 Popliteal artery
3 Arcuate artery with dorsal metatarsal arteries
4 Plantar arch
5 Posterior tibial artery
6 Anterior tibial artery
7 Fibular (peroneal) artery
8 Femoral artery

Description:

Continued from page 56

Arteries are flexible, thick-walled tubes that carry blood under pressure away from the heart to the rest of the body. From the arteries, blood passes into capillaries—the smallest type of blood vessel in the vascular system—and from there, blood passes to veins and then back to the heart. The heart also pumps blood through the pulmonary artery to the lungs, where it becomes oxygenated and loses carbon dioxide. The blood is then returned to the heart, where it is once again pumped out through the aorta.

anterior view

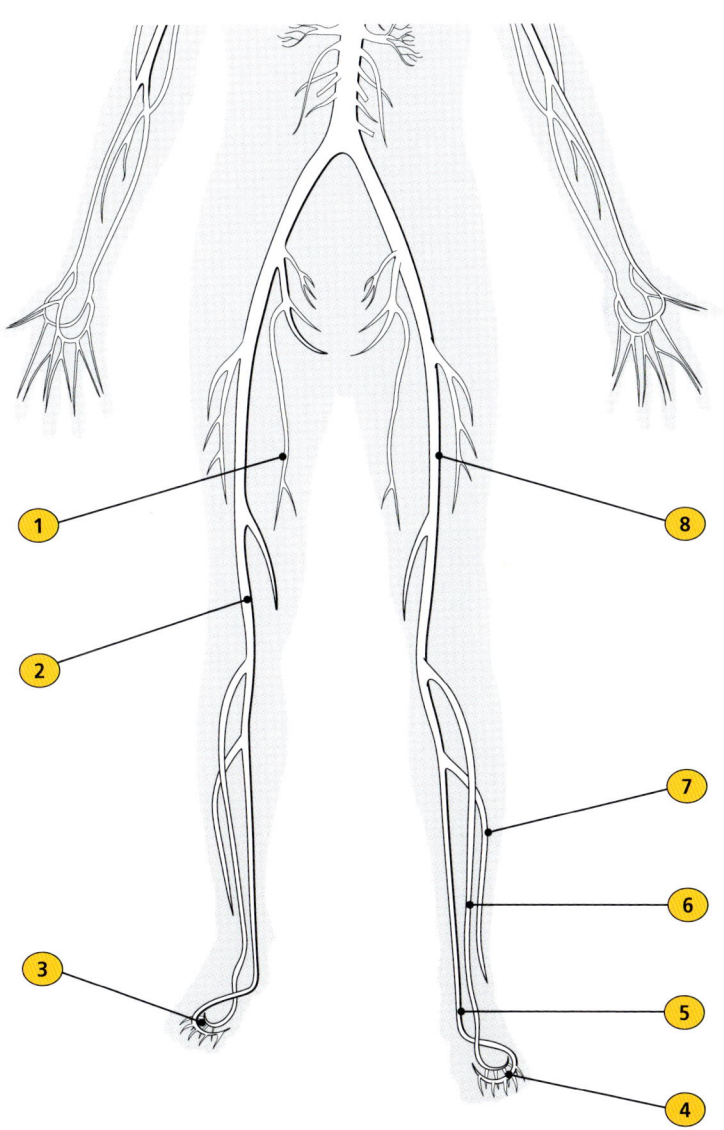

Major Veins of the Circulatory System

Key:

1	External jugular vein	**10**	Palmar venous arch
2	Internal jugular vein	**11**	Ulnar vein
3	Axillary vein	**12**	Radial vein
4	Cephalic vein	**13**	Inferior vena cava
5	Azygos vein	**14**	Renal vein
6	Brachial vein	**15**	Superior vena cava
7	Basilic vein	**16**	Subclavian vein
8	Median cubital vein	**17**	Brachiocephalic vein
9	Common iliac vein		

Description:

The two largest veins in the body are the superior and inferior vena cavae, which drain into the heart from above and below, respectively.

The brachial, basilic, and cephalic veins drain the upper limbs into the axillary vein, which becomes the subclavian vein. The internal jugular vein, which drains the head and brain, joins the subclavian vein to form the brachiocephalic vein. The left and right brachiocephalic veins join to form the superior vena cava, which drains into the heart. The azygos vein, which drains the thoracic cavity, joins the superior vena cava.

Continued on page 62

anterior view

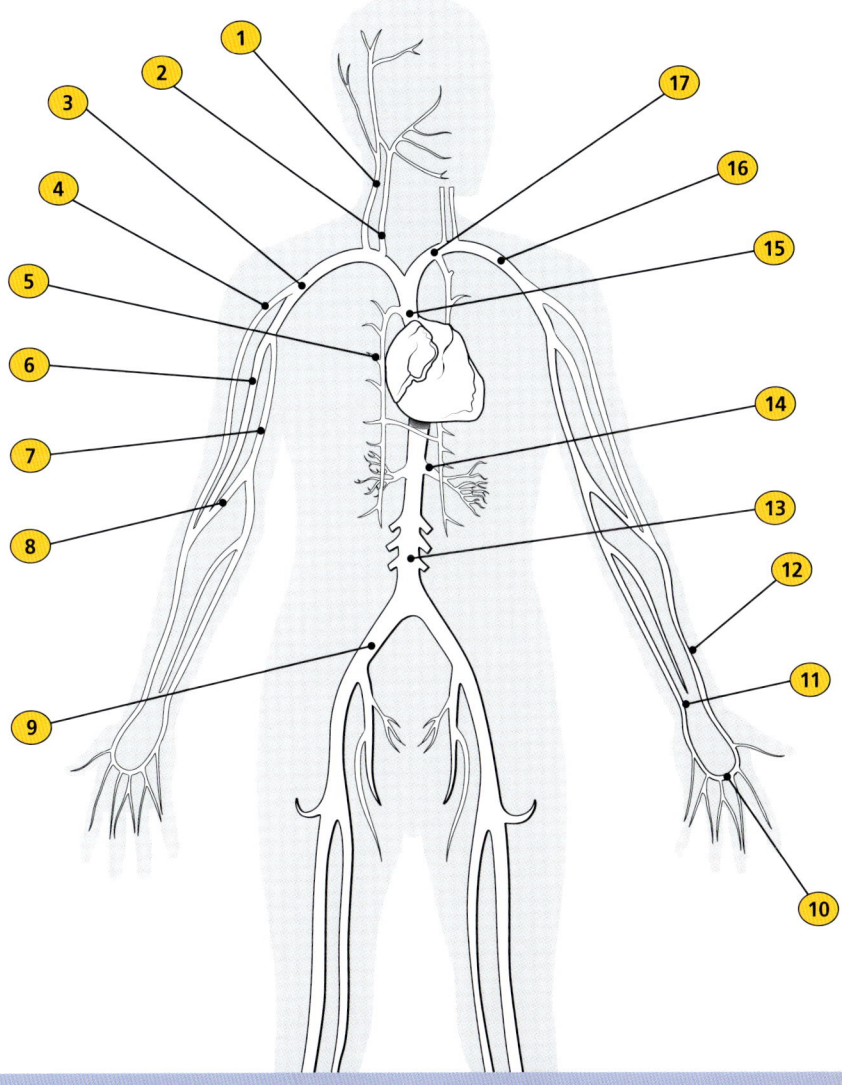

Major Veins of the Circulatory System

Key:

1 Femoral vein
2 Obturator vein
3 Plantar venous arch
4 Dorsal venous arch
5 Great saphenous vein
6 Small saphenous vein
7 Popliteal vein
8 External iliac vein
9 Internal iliac vein

Description:

Continued from page 60

The femoral vein drains the lower limb, becoming the external iliac vein as it enters the trunk. It is joined by the internal iliac vein to become the common iliac vein. The common iliac veins join to form the inferior vena cava. It joins with veins from the kidneys, gonads, liver, and back region, passes through the diaphragm, and enters the heart.

Note: The small saphenous vein has been deliberately displaced laterally for illustrative reasons and usually runs up the posterior surface of the calf.

anterior view

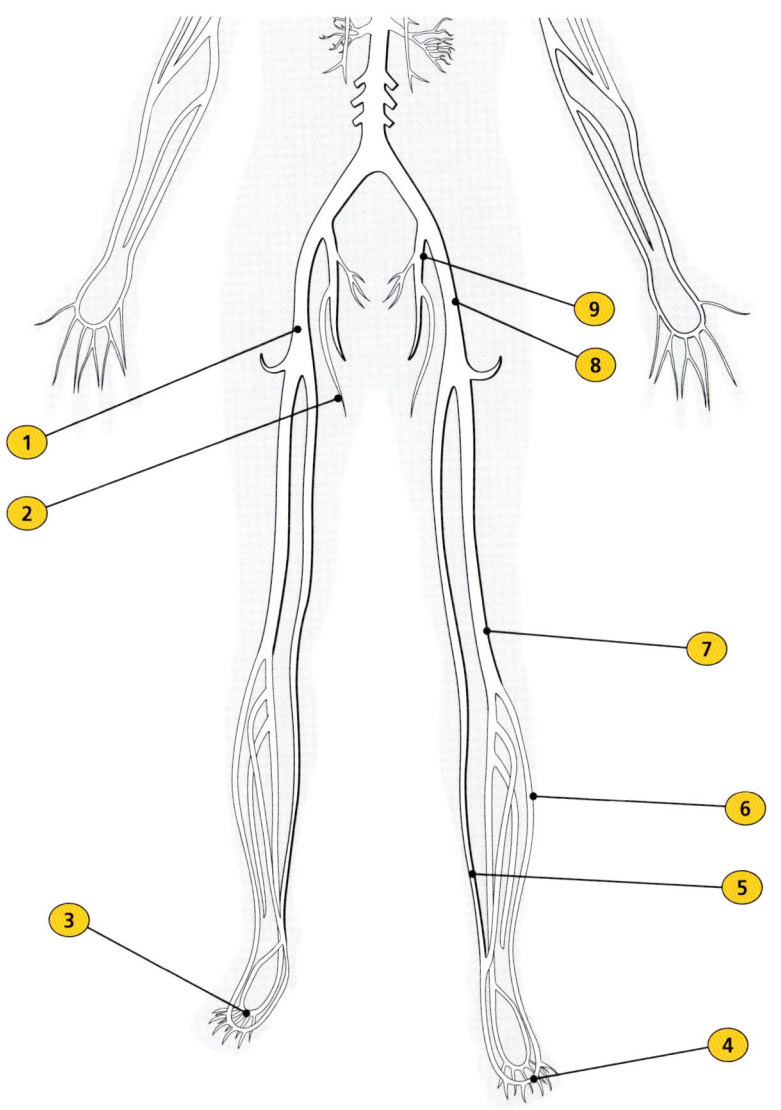

Cerebral Arteries

Key:

1 Anterior communicating artery
2 Internal carotid artery
3 Posterior cerebral artery
4 Basilar artery
5 Anterior inferior cerebellar artery
6 Posterior inferior cerebellar artery
7 Vertebral artery
8 Labyrinthine artery
9 Superior cerebellar artery
10 Posterior communicating artery
11 Middle cerebral artery (hidden behind temporal lobe)
12 Anterior cerebral artery

Description:
The brain is supplied by a network of arteries known as the cerebral arteries. The cerebral arteries are formed from the carotid and vertebral arteries. The carotid arteries supply the front (anterior cerebral arteries) and middle (middle cerebral arteries) of the brain—the vertebral arteries supply the back of the brain, cerebellum, and brainstem (posterior cerebral and cerebellar arteries). The three paired cerebral arteries (anterior, middle, and posterior) are joined by communicating arteries (anterior and posterior) to form the cerebral arterial circle (of Willis). The labyrinthine artery supplies the inner ear.

inferior view

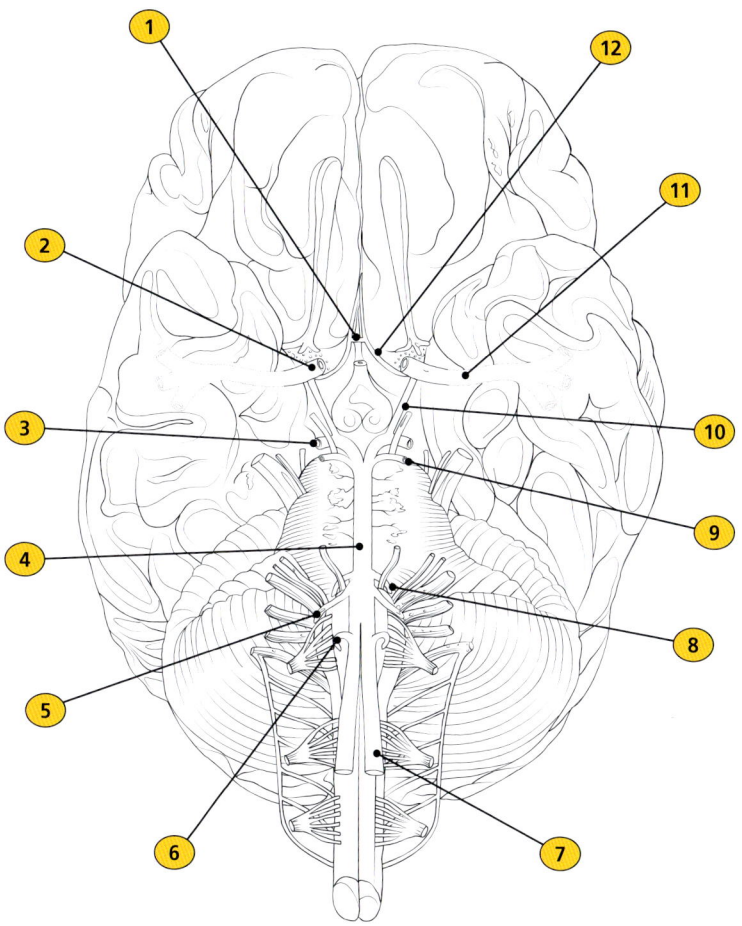

Cerebral Arteries

Key:

1 Paracentral artery
2 Pericallosal artery
3 Medial frontal branches (of callosomarginal artery)
4 Callosomarginal artery
5 Polar frontal artery
6 Medial frontobasal artery
7 Medial striate artery
8 Right anterior cerebral artery
9 Posterior cerebral artery
10 Calcarine branch (of medial occipital artery)
11 Parietooccipital branch (of medial occipital artery)
12 Medial occipital artery
13 Precuneal artery

Description:

The anterior cerebral artery has many branches and is itself one of the terminal branches of the internal carotid artery. This network of branches supplies blood to the various parts of the brain and anterior forebrain, including the corpus callosum and the frontal lobes of the brain. The posterior cerebral artery is an essential artery for supply of the primary visual cortex (calcarine branch). Although the brain makes up only 2 percent of the average body weight, it uses 20 percent of the available oxygen.

sagittal view

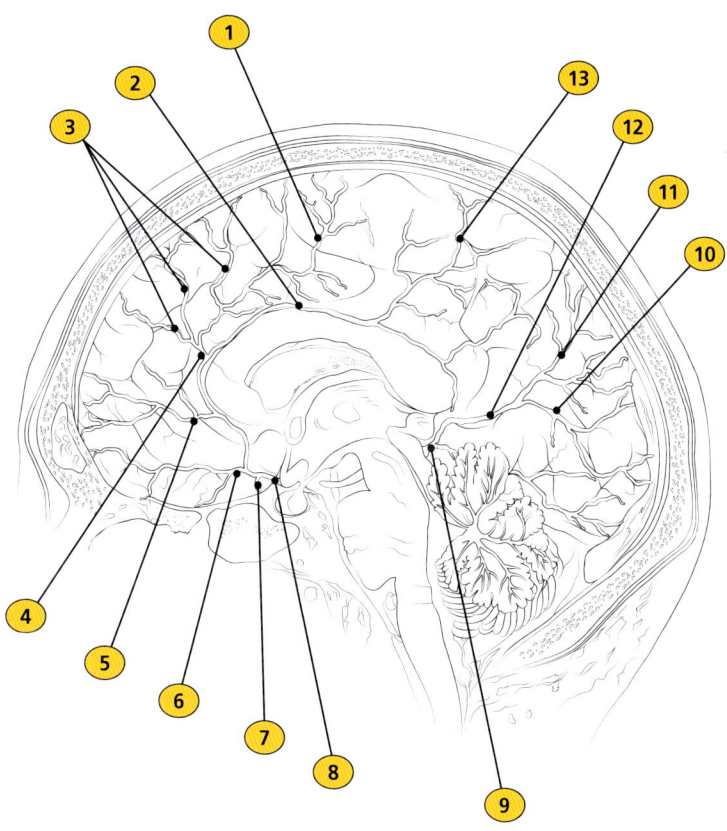

Circulatory System

Superficial Arteries of the Head and Neck

Key:

1. Supraorbital artery
2. Supratrochlear artery
3. Transverse facial artery
4. Facial artery
5. Transverse cervical artery
6. External carotid artery
7. Superficial temporal artery
8. Occipital artery
9. Anterior branch of superficial temporal artery
10. Posterior branch of superficial temporal artery

Description:

The superficial blood vessels of the head and neck are supplied by branches of the external carotid artery, which lie on each side of the neck. Numerous branches lead away from the external carotid artery, supplying blood to the neck, skull, and face. The branches include: the superficial temporal artery, which extends to the top of the head; the facial artery, which extends across the cheek area to the medial side of the eye; the occipital artery, which extends behind the ear; and the deeper maxillary artery (not shown), which supplies the jaw, nose, and teeth.

lateral view

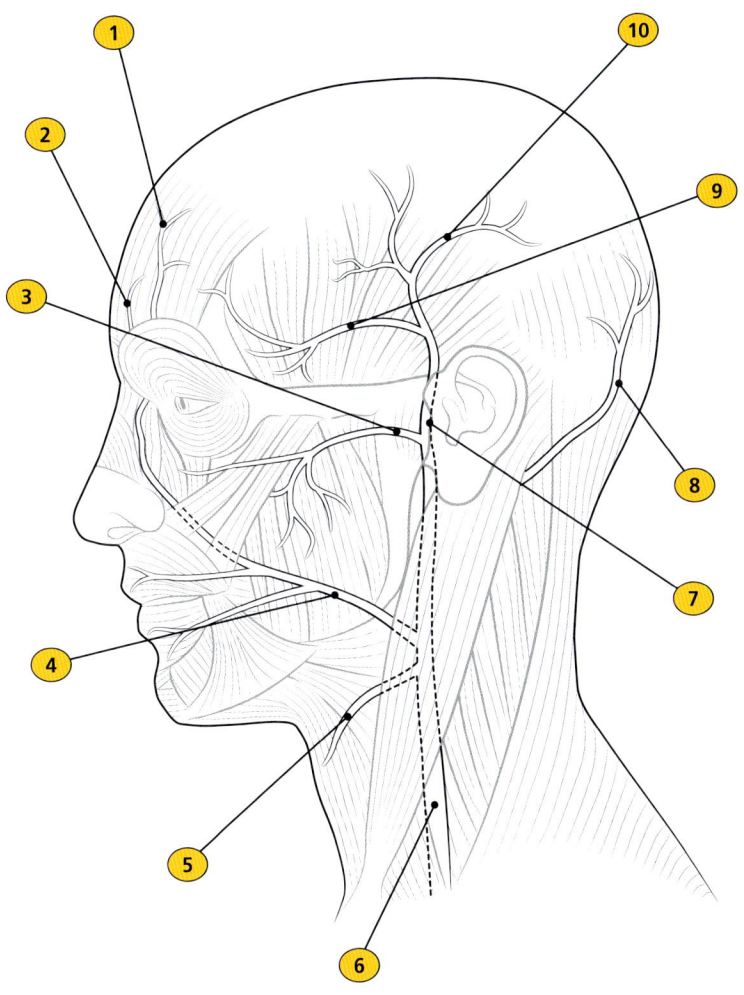

Superficial Veins of the Head and Neck

Key:

1 Anterior branch of superficial temporal vein
2 Supraorbital vein
3 Supratrochlear vein
4 Facial vein
5 Submental vein
6 Internal jugular vein
7 Brachiocephalic vein
8 Subclavian vein
9 External jugular vein
10 Retromandibular vein
11 Posterior auricular vein
12 Occipital vein
13 Posterior branch of superficial temporal vein

Description:
The principal superficial veins of the head and neck are the temporal, facial, and occipital veins. These veins drain the superficial area above, in front of, and behind the ear, respectively; the area around the cheeks and nose; and the area around the jaw. These veins drain into the external jugular veins that lie on each side of the neck. Blood from the external jugular veins is then carried back to the heart.

lateral view

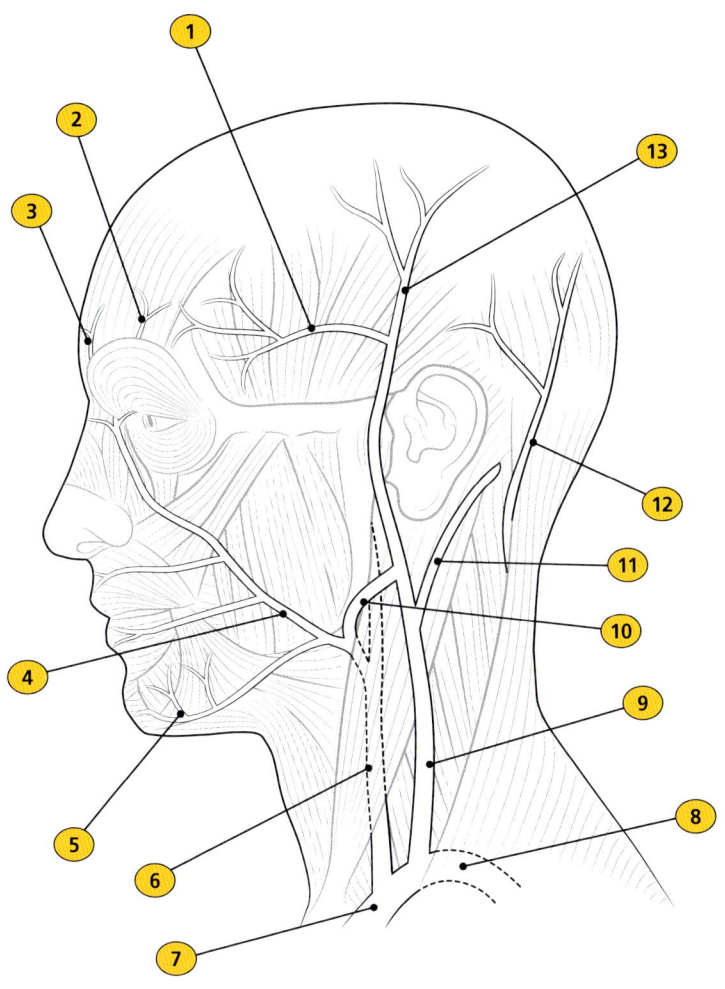

Circulatory System

Blood Vessels of the Eye

Key:

1 Minor arterial circle
2 Major arterial circle
3 Choriocapillaris
4 Central vein of retina
5 Central artery of retina
6 Long posterior ciliary artery
7 Short posterior ciliary artery
8 Vorticose vein

Description:

The central artery of the retina enters the eyeball after running through the center of the optic nerve. As it emerges from the optic disk, the central artery of the retina fans out into four main branches accompanied by their veins. These branches run on the inside of the retina and spread out into the capillary network.

The central vein of the retina receives blood from the retinal veins. Blood from the central vein of the retina drains into the superior ophthalmic vein.

lateral view

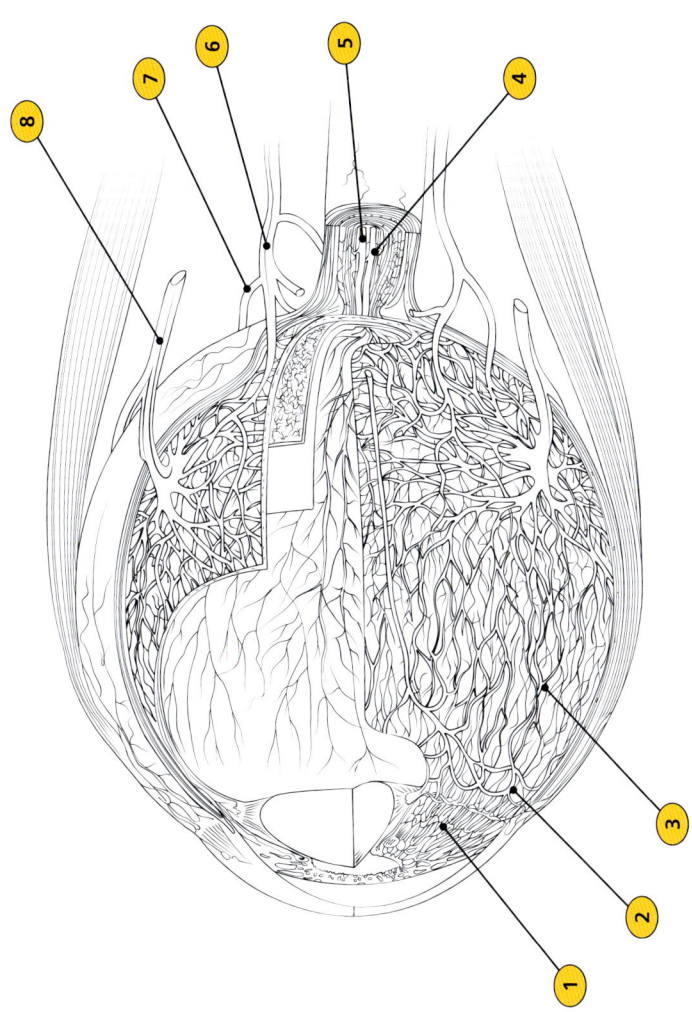

Circulatory System

Heart and Lungs

Key:

1	Left brachiocephalic vein	**11**	Right lung (lower lobe)
2	Brachiocephalic trunk	**12**	Pleura
3	Right common carotid artery	**13**	Right ventricle
		14	Diaphragm
4	Right subclavian artery	**15**	Left ventricle
5	Right brachiocephalic vein	**16**	Pulmonary trunk
6	Right lung (upper lobe)	**17**	Left pulmonary artery
7	Ascending aorta	**18**	Left lung (upper lobe)
8	Superior vena cava	**19**	Aortic arch
9	Pericardium	**20**	Left subclavian artery
10	Right atrium	**21**	Left common carotid artery

Description:

The heart and lungs are components of the thorax—the body region lying below the neck, and separated from the abdomen by the diaphragm—with the ribs encircling the thorax for protection. The heart lies in the midline of the thorax, between the lungs. These two organs work together in the circulatory system.

There are two separate circuits in the circulatory system, which are connected in a series—the systemic circulation and the pulmonary circulation. In the systemic circulation, blood from the left ventricle is distributed to the capillaries through the body to deliver oxygen and nutrients to the entire body. Veins return the deoxygenated blood to the right atrium. This blood is also loaded with carbon dioxide. The blood flows into the right ventricle, where it is pumped into the pulmonary circulation including the capillary network in the lungs. Carbon dioxide is exchanged with oxygen, and the oxygenated blood returns to the left atrium.

anterior view

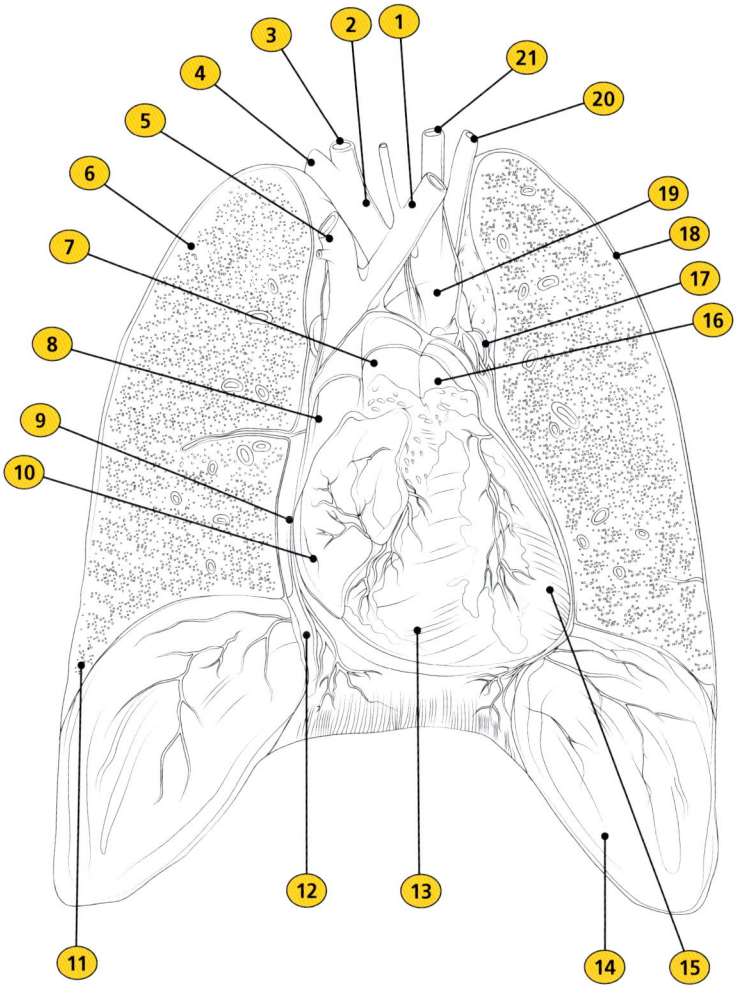

Arterial System of the Abdomen

Key:

1	Pancreaticoduodenal artery	10	Superior mesenteric artery
2	Right colic artery	11	Splenic artery
3	Ileocolic artery	12	Gastroduodenal artery
4	Appendicular artery	13	Common hepatic artery
5	Rectal artery	14	Celiac trunk
6	Sigmoidal artery	15	Hepatic artery proper
7	Jejunal and ileal arteries	16	Thoracic aorta
8	Inferior mesenteric artery	17	Inferior vena cava
9	Left colic artery		

Description:

The gastrointestinal tract is supplied by unpaired anterior branches of the abdominal aorta (celiac trunk and superior and inferior mesenteric arteries).

The celiac artery supplies the stomach, liver, gallbladder, spleen, proximal duodenum, and pancreas. The superior mesenteric artery supplies the distal duodenum, jejunum, ileum, cecum, appendix, and ascending and transverse colon. The inferior mesenteric artery supplies the descending and sigmoid colon, and the rectum as far as the pectinate line. The kidneys, adrenals, gonads, and pelvic organs are supplied by paired lateral branches of the abdominal aorta (the suprarenal, renal, and ovarian or testicular arteries) and iliac vessels.

anterior view

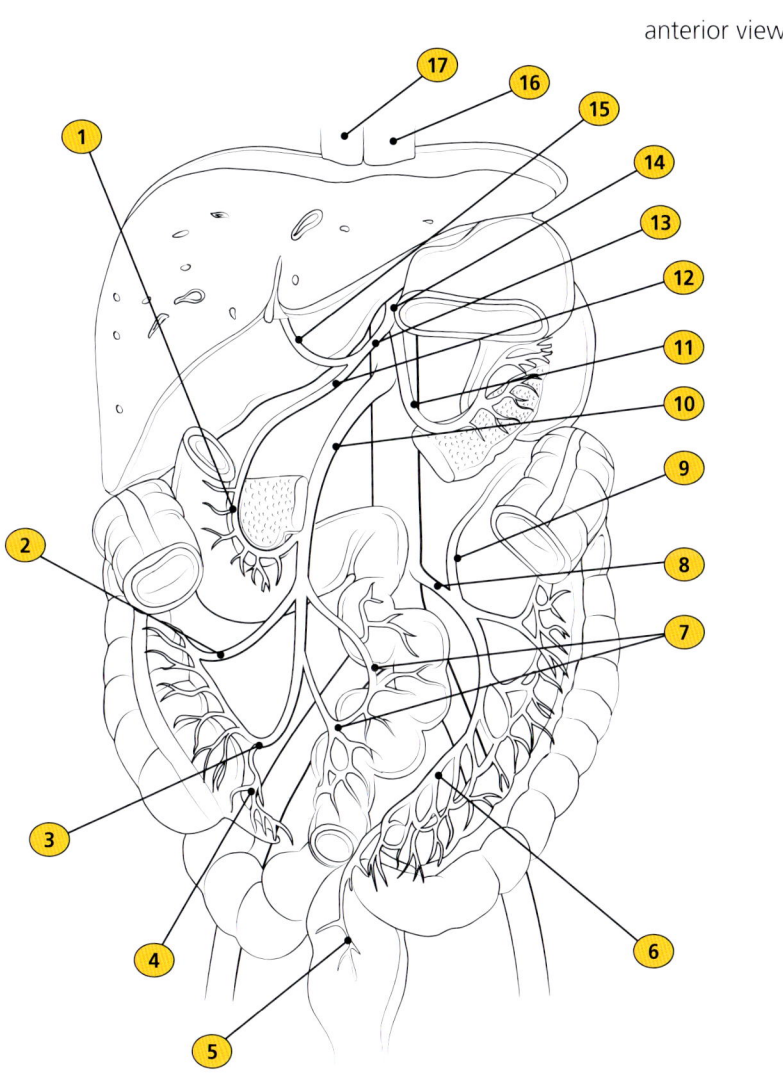

Portal System

Key:

1	Inferior vena cava	**11**	Small intestine
2	Liver	**12**	Left colic veins
3	Portal vein	**13**	Inferior mesenteric vein
4	Duodenum	**14**	Pancreas
5	Pancreaticoduodenal vein	**15**	Splenic vein
6	Superior mesenteric vein	**16**	Spleen
7	Right colic vein	**17**	Left gastric vein
8	Appendicular vein	**18**	Stomach
9	Colon	**19**	Thoracic aorta
10	Rectum		

Description:

Nutrients extracted during the digestive process are delivered to the liver via numerous blood vessels that converge at the portal vein. Blood carrying nutrients and a small amount of waste products and toxins enters the portal venous system serving the intestine, the major components of which are the superior and inferior mesenteric veins and the splenic vein.

The inferior mesenteric vein frequently joins the splenic vein, which drains the accessory digestive organs of the pancreas and spleen, as well as part of the stomach. The inferior mesenteric vein may join the superior mesenteric vein. The superior mesenteric and splenic veins join to form the portal vein. The left gastric vein, which drains the upper part of the stomach, and the cystic veins, which drain the gallbladder, also drain into the portal vein. Once blood delivered by the hepatic portal system has filtered through the liver, it is returned to the heart via the inferior vena cava.

anterior view

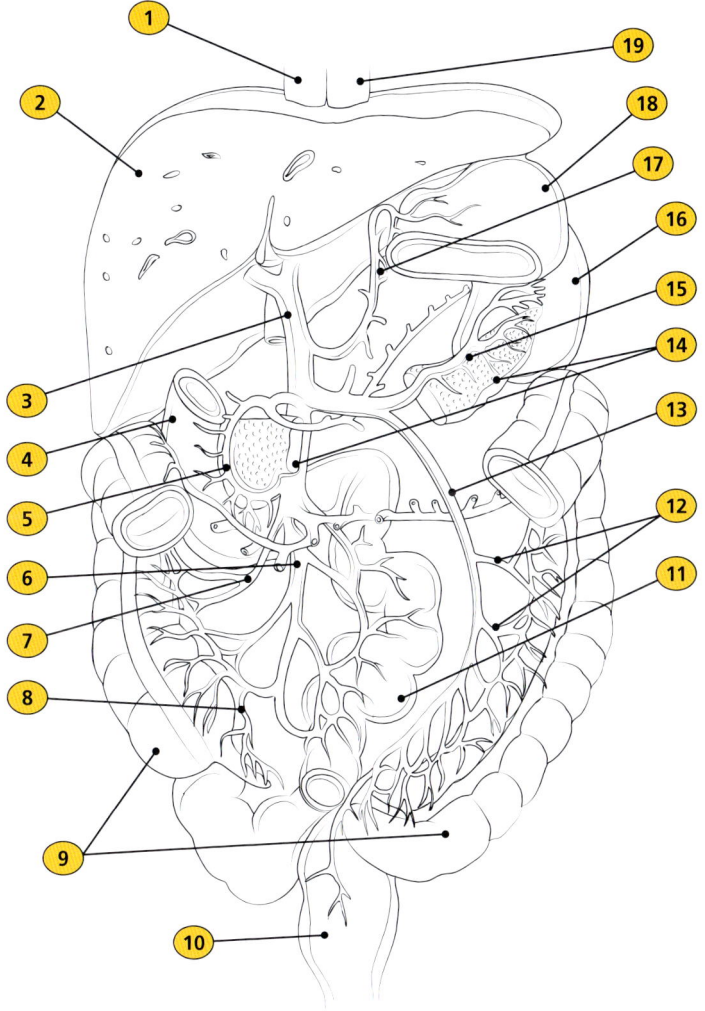

Renal Arteries

Key:

1 Celiac trunk	**8** Segmental artery
2 Superior mesenteric artery	**9** Arcuate artery
3 Left renal artery	**10** Interlobar artery
4 Right gonadal artery	**11** Renal pyramid (medulla)
5 Left gonadal artery	**12** Cortex
6 Abdominal aorta	**13** Left adrenal gland
7 Ureter	

Description:

The renal arteries are two large blood vessels that branch off either side of the abdominal aorta to supply the two kidneys. Near each kidney, each renal artery divides into segmental arteries, which enter the hilum of a kidney, where each artery then gives off small branches to the adrenal gland and ureter, and then divides into two large branches—the anterior and posterior divisions of the artery. Each branch then divides into smaller and smaller branches, eventually forming the capillaries that supply oxygen to the kidneys and take part in kidney filtration via their role in the kidney nephrons.

anterior view with coronal cross-section—left kidney

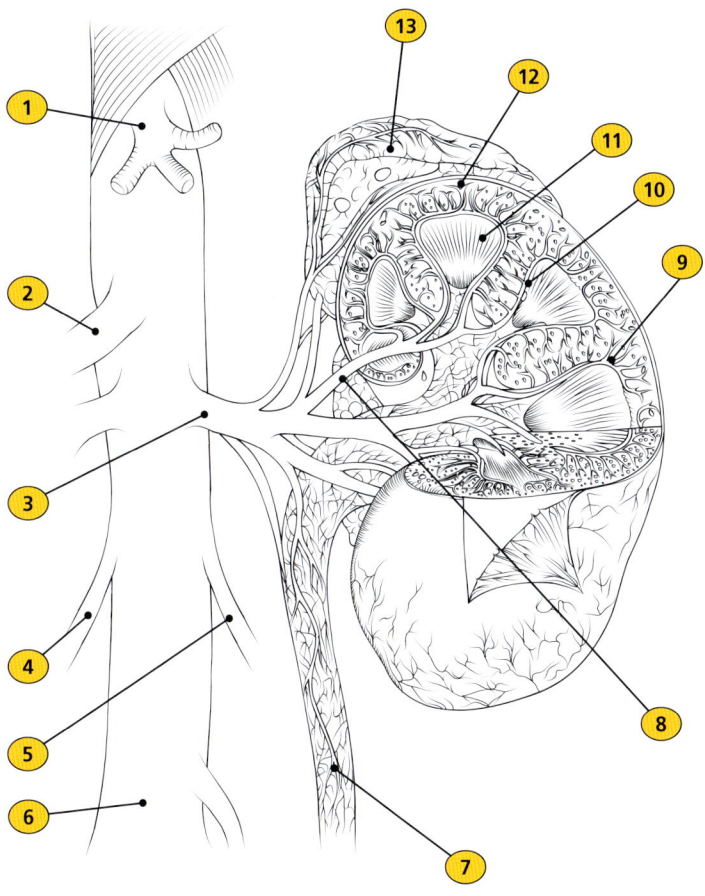

Arteries of the Pelvic Wall: Female

Key:

1 Common iliac artery
2 Internal iliac artery
3 External iliac artery
4 Obturator artery
5 Obliterated umbilical artery
6 Superior vesical arteries
7 Uterine artery

8 Vaginal artery
9 Middle rectal artery
10 Internal pudendal artery
11 Inferior gluteal artery
12 Superior gluteal artery
13 Lateral sacral artery
14 Iliolumbar artery

Description:

Blood is supplied to the pelvis by the right and left internal iliac arteries arising from the respective common iliac arteries. The arrangement of branches is variable, but typically the divisions are posterior (to the pelvic wall structures) and anterior (to the pelvic organs and the gluteal and perineal regions). The pelvic arteries include branches to pelvic viscera (uterine and vaginal arteries in females, inferior vesical arteries in males) and branches to the body wall (gluteal, lateral sacral, and iliolumbar arteries). The internal pudendal artery supplies the anal canal and external genitalia.

lateral view—right pelvic cavity

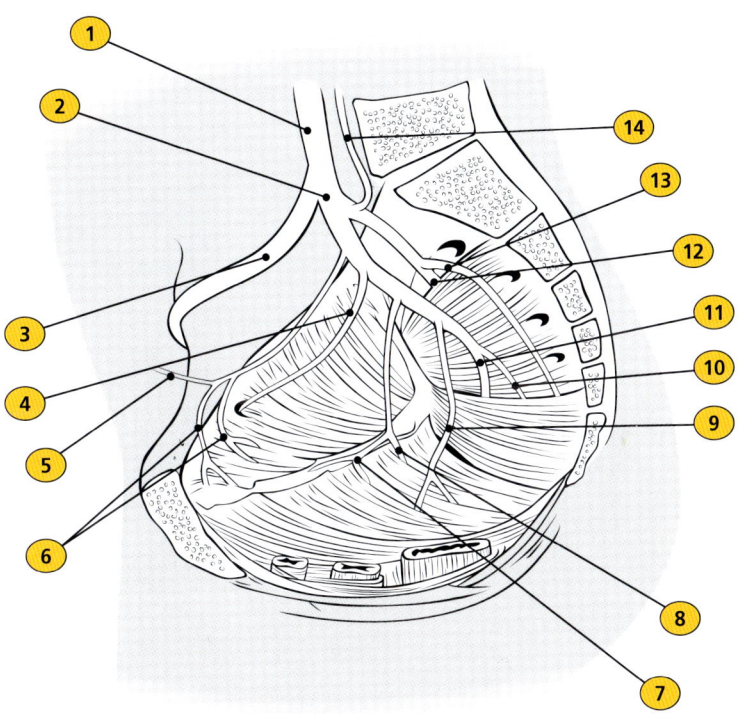

Arteries of the Upper Limb

Key:

1 Lateral thoracic artery
2 Subscapular artery
3 Brachial artery
4 Superior ulnar collateral artery
5 Ulnar artery
6 Deep palmar arch
7 Common palmar digital arteries

8 Superficial palmar arch
9 Radial artery
10 Interosseous artery
11 Deep brachial artery
12 Axillary artery
13 Subclavian artery

Description:

A continuation of the axillary artery, the brachial artery is the major artery of the upper limb. It runs down the length of the arm, dividing at the elbow into two major branches—the radial artery and the ulnar artery—that supply the forearm and hand. There are additional collateral arteries around the elbow. The radial artery is often used as a pulse point. The radial and ulnar arteries contribute to palmar arches which branch to form common palmar digital arteries and then distal digital arteries in the fingers.

anterior view—left limb

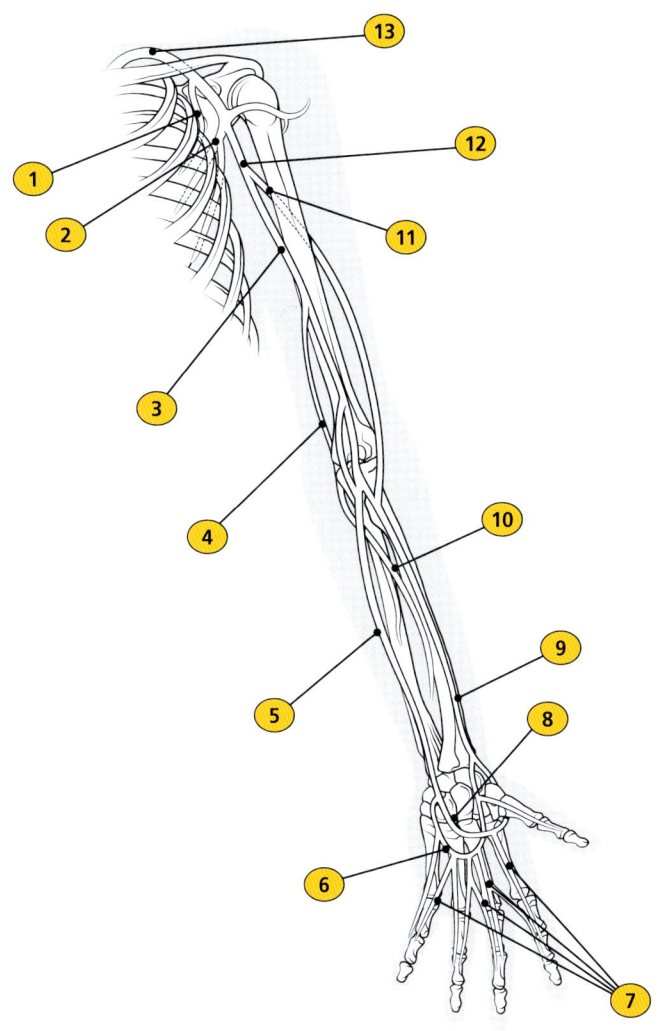

Veins of the Upper Limb

Key:

1 Brachial vein
2 Basilic vein
3 Median cubital vein
4 Median antebrachial vein
5 Palmar venous arch
6 Digital veins
7 Cephalic vein
8 Axillary vein
9 Subclavian vein

Description:

In the upper limb, the veins are organized into two groups—the deep group and the superficial group. The deep-group veins travel with the deep arteries and are similarly named. The superficial-group veins travel immediately beneath the skin. Returning blood to the heart, the network of veins in the arm drains into the axillary vein. Blood from the superficial palmar venous arch drains into the cephalic and basilic veins. The basilic vein joins up with the brachial vein and, along with the cephalic vein, drains into the axillary vein.

anterior view—left limb

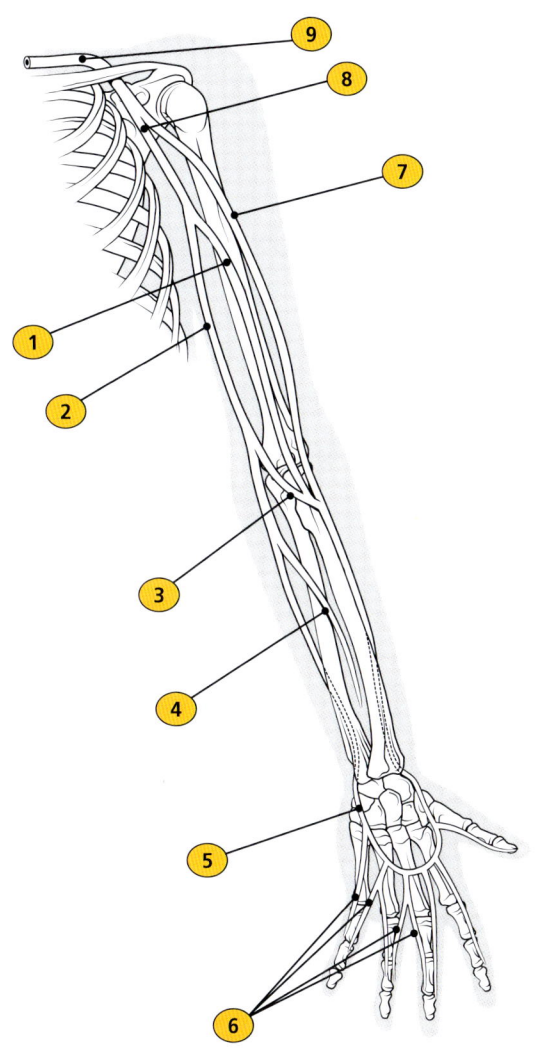

Circulatory System

Arteries of the Lower Limb

Key:

1 Femoral artery
2 Obturator artery
3 Descending genicular artery
4 Posterior tibial artery
5 Arcuate artery
6 Plantar arch
7 Fibular (peroneal) artery
8 Anterior tibial artery
9 Popliteal artery
10 Deep femoral artery

Description:
Most of the blood supplied to the lower limbs travels from the aorta to the external iliac artery. This becomes the femoral artery as it enters the thigh by passing deep to the inguinal ligament at the groin. Two-thirds of the way down the thigh, the femoral artery passes backward through the adductor canal and passes behind the knee to become the popliteal artery. The popliteal artery then divides into anterior and posterior tibial branches that descend in the anterior and posterior compartments of the lower part of the leg, before entering the foot.

The posterior tibial artery branches into medial and lateral plantar arteries which in turn contribute to superficial and deep plantar arches. Plantar metatarsal arteries arise from the plantar arches and branch to form plantar digital arteries.

anterior view—left limb

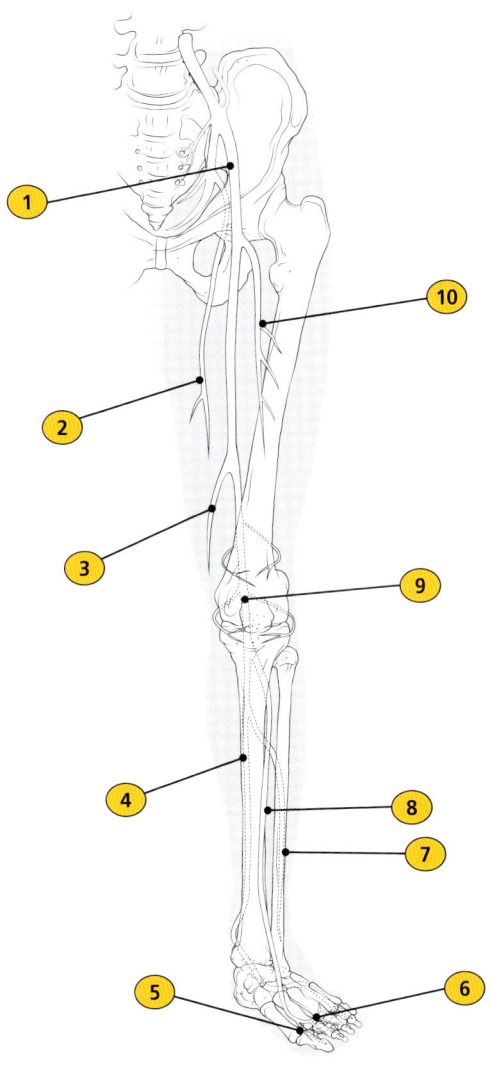

Veins of the Lower Limb

Key:
1 External iliac vein
2 Obturator vein
3 Great saphenous vein
4 Anterior tibial vein
5 Posterior tibial vein
6 Dorsal venous arch
7 Digital veins
8 Plantar venous arch
9 Small saphenous vein
10 Fibular (peroneal) vein
11 Femoral vein

Description:
The veins of the lower limb are organized into two groups of veins—the deep group and the superficial group. The members of the deep group of lower limb veins travel with the deep arteries and are similarly named. The superficial veins, such as the great and small saphenous veins, travel in the superficial tissue just below the skin. Lower limb veins have numerous valves directing blood toward the heart. Compression of veins by calf muscles helps to pump blood back toward the heart.

Note: The small saphenous vein has been deliberately displaced laterally for illustrative reasons and usually runs up the posterior surface of the calf.

anterior view—left limb

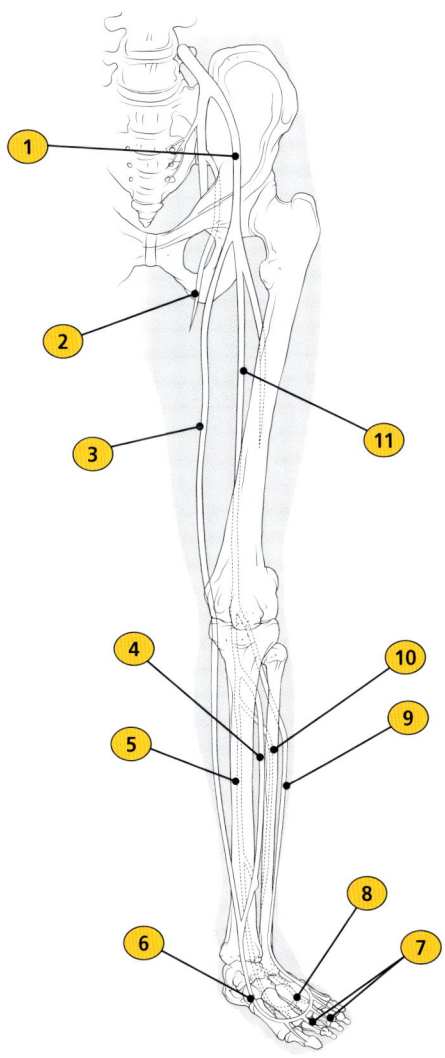

Lymphatic System

Not all the fluid that leaves the heart in the systemic arteries is returned to the heart by the veins. This small amount of excess fluid from the capillary beds is drained from the tissue spaces by the lymphatic system and is eventually returned to the systemic veins. The lymphatic drainage passes through chains of lymph nodes that monitor the tissue fluid for the presence of foreign substances, microorganisms, or cancer cells, and can signal the cells of the immune system (neutrophils, macrophages, plasma cells, lymphocytes) to begin a defensive response against foreign invaders and cancer cells.

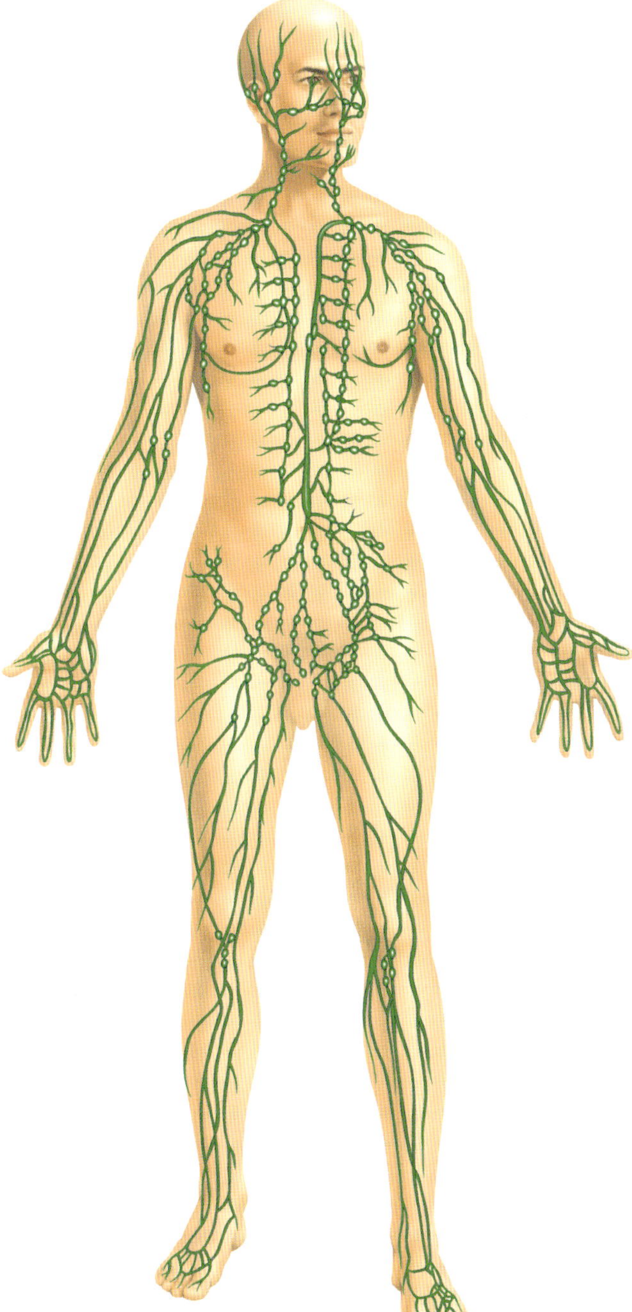

Lymphatic System

Key:

1	Retroauricular nodes	**10**	Sacral nodes
2	Parotid nodes	**11**	External iliac nodes
3	Axillary nodes	**12**	Common iliac nodes
4	Apical axillary nodes	**13**	Cisterna chyli
5	Lateral group	**14**	Posterior mediastinal nodes
6	Anterior group	**15**	Thoracic duct
7	Parasternal nodes	**16**	Cervical nodes
8	Posterior intercostal nodes	**17**	Buccal nodes
9	Cubital nodes		

Description:

The lymphatic system, a network of vessels and aggregates of lymphoid tissue (lymph nodes and tonsils), has two main functions. Apart from bringing back to the heart much of the interstitial fluid that bathes all cells of the body, it is also loaded with lymphocytes and macrophages, which sweep up foreign bodies or invaders, such as bacteria, viruses, and cancer cells.

The lymphatic system is a one-way system that begins with a capillary-like network of blind-ended tubes. These capillaries collect large molecules and particles (foreign bodies and nutritional elements) and water (interstitial fluid), and converge to form gradually larger lymphatic vessels that carry the lymph toward the heart.

Continued on page 96

anterior view

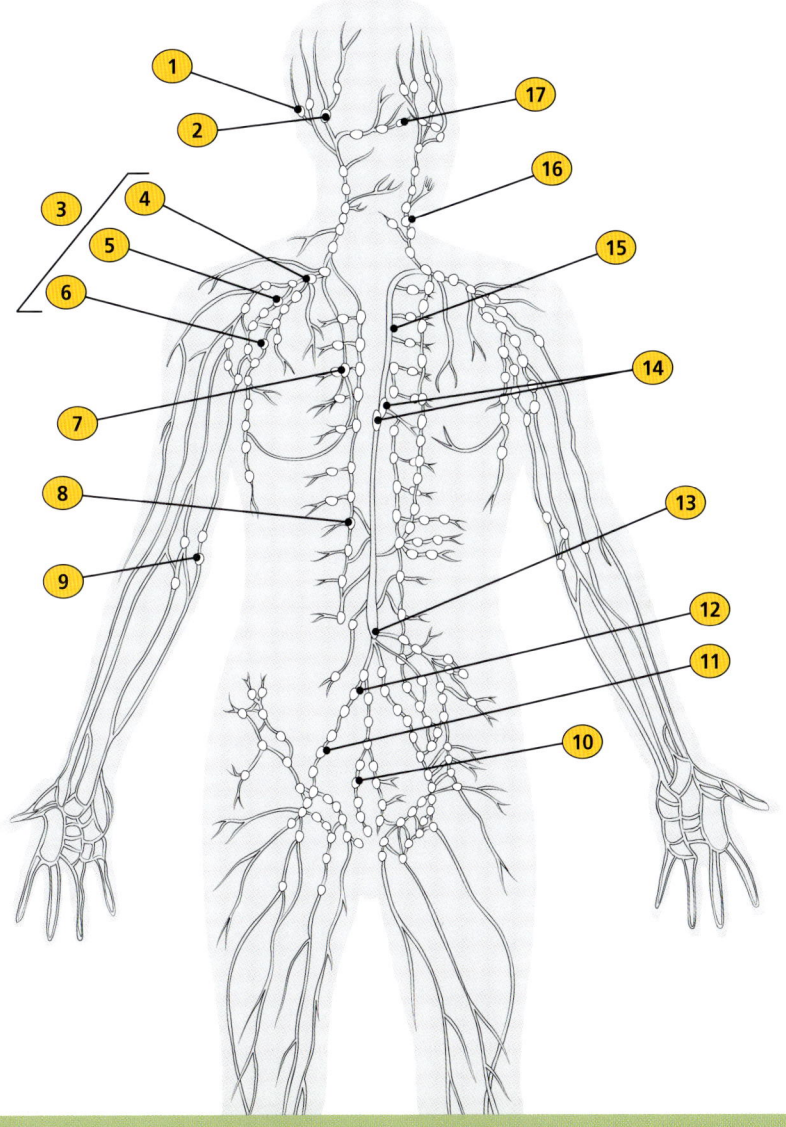

Lymphatic System

Key:

   1 Palmar and dorsal plexus
   2 Plantar and dorsal plexus
   3 Popliteal nodes (posterior side of the knee)
   4 Inguinal and femoral nodes

Description:

Continued from page 94

Lymph vessels form a parallel circulation to the veins and arteries through the body. Lymph vessels have valves to ensure one-way flow. Collections of lymph nodes (frequently and colloquially called lymph glands) are found along the lymph vessels. The lymph nodes are small pea-sized organs located in groups at the confluence of lymphatic vessels. Each lymph node is connected to incoming and outgoing lymphatic vessels. Incoming lymph percolates through the lymph node to pass through aggregations of lymphocytes and macrophages. Debris or foreign matter and cancer cells are engulfed by macrophages and specialized lymphocytes called killer cells.

   Lymph nodes also activate the cloning of lymphocytes to produce specific antibodies to antigens in bacteria, which is part of the immune response. Lymphoid tissue, exemplified by the tonsils, is made up of collections of lymphocytes and other cells that monitor immunity around the mouth and along the wall of the gastrointestinal tract.

Lymphatic System

anterior view

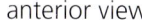

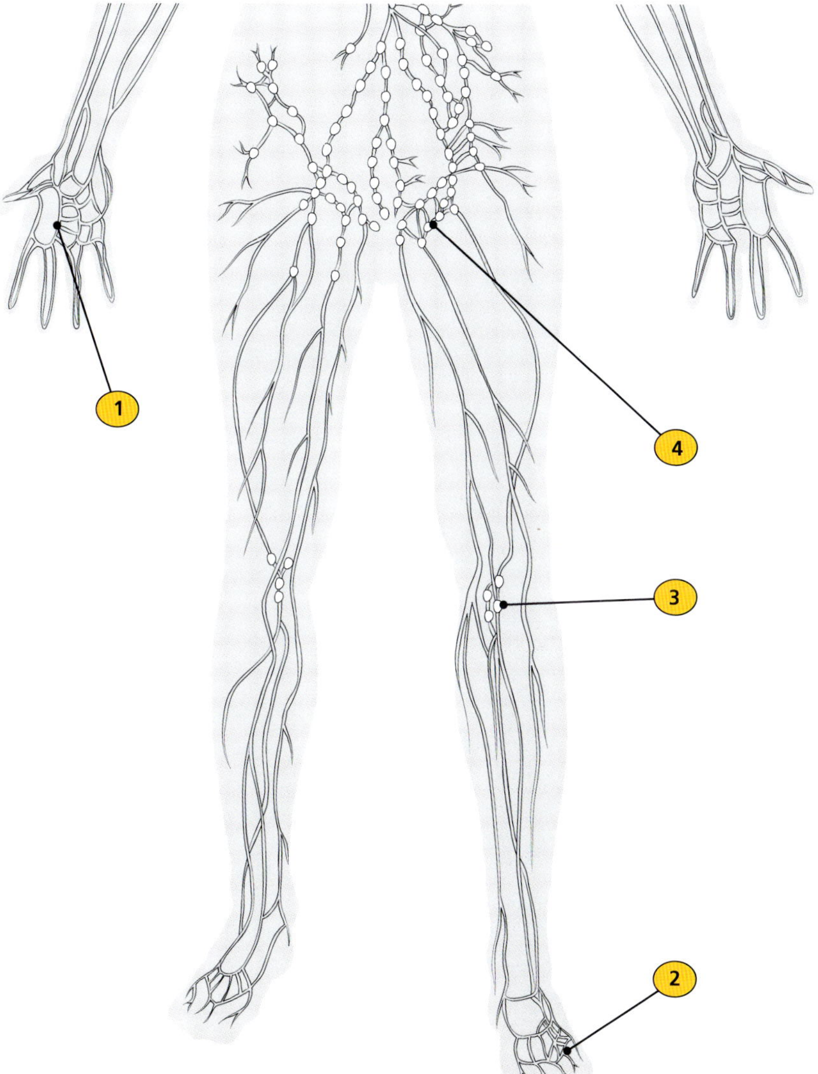

1

2

3

4

Lymph Node

Key:

1 Medullary sinus
2 Follicle of cortex
3 Blood capillary
4 Valve
5 Efferent lymphatic vessel
6 Artery
7 Vein
8 Subcapsular sinus
9 Capsule
10 Trabeculae
11 Afferent lymphatic vessels

Description:

Lymph is a fluid that is filtered and cleaned by white blood cells in the lymph nodes (glands). A lymph node consists of a mass of lymphatic tissue that is surrounded by a fibrous capsule. The nodes cluster in groups along the lymphatic vessels. Each node is enclosed in a fibrous capsule and has compartments divided by partitions of collagen fibers (trabeculae).

Each lymph node is connected to incoming and outgoing lymph vessels. Afferent lymphatic vessels bring lymph fluid to the node from surrounding tissues; efferent vessels transport lymph to the veins. Numerous valves prevent the backflow of lymph as it passes through the lymphatic vessels.

cross-sectional view

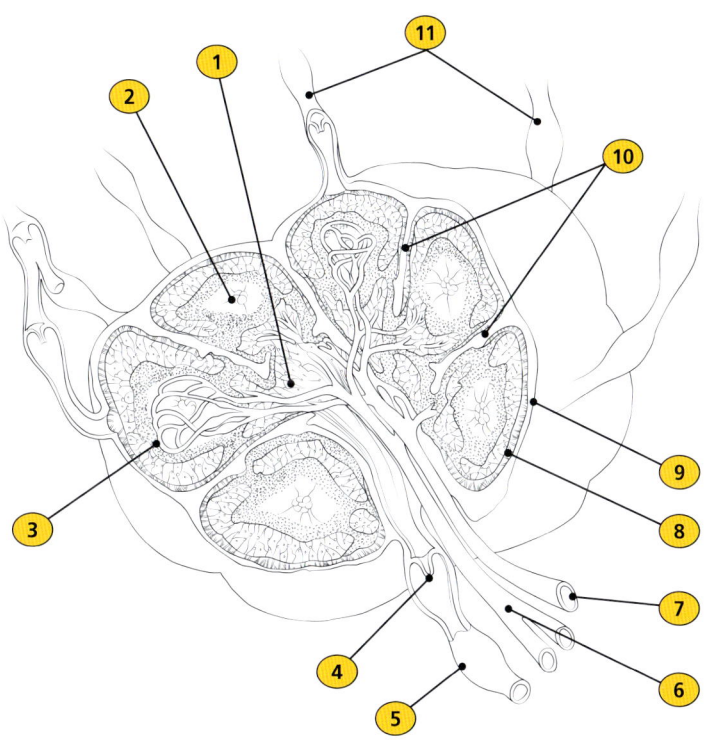

Lymphoid Organs of the Head

Key:
- **1** Lingual tonsil
- **2** Palatine tonsil
- **3** Pharyngeal tonsil (adenoid)

Description:

The tonsils are lymphoid organs that lie under the surface lining of the mouth and throat. There are three sets of tonsils, named according to their position. The lingual tonsil lies on the back third of the tongue; the palatine tonsils lie on either side of the back of the tongue, between pillars of tissue that join the soft palate to the tongue; and the pharyngeal or nasopharyngeal tonsils (adenoids) lie in the space behind the nose.

The tonsils are arranged around the entrance to the respiratory and digestive tracts to protect the body from bacteria and viruses that may enter from the mouth and nose. The tonsils produce lymphocytes, which cross into the mouth and throat.

sagittal view

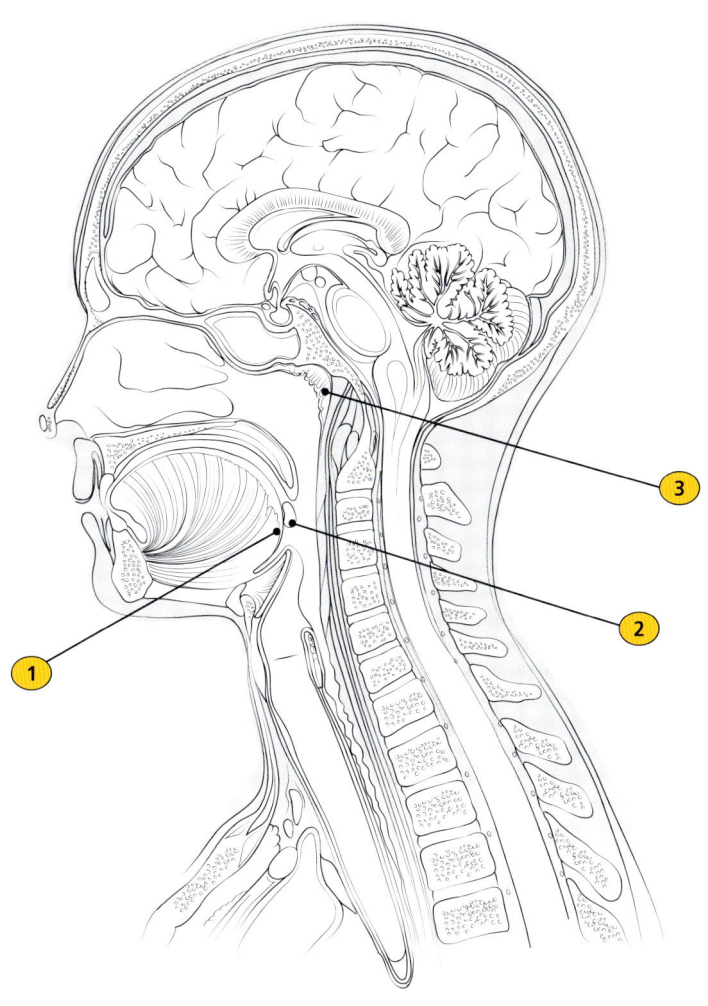

Thymus

Key:

1 Right lobe
2 Left lobe

Description:

The thymus lies in the upper part of the thorax, between the heart and the sternum. It is the first lymphoid organ to develop in the embryo, and reaches 1–1½ ounces (30–40 g) at puberty. It is gradually replaced by fat and fibrous tissue after puberty.

The thymus produces T lymphocytes for distribution to the body. T lymphocytes divide in the cortex of the thymus, moving into the medulla when mature. These T cells leave the thymus after about three weeks, entering the body's circulation via the blood vessels. When the thymus regresses after puberty, T cells continue to proliferate in other lymphoid organs, thus maintaining an adequate number throughout life.

anterior view

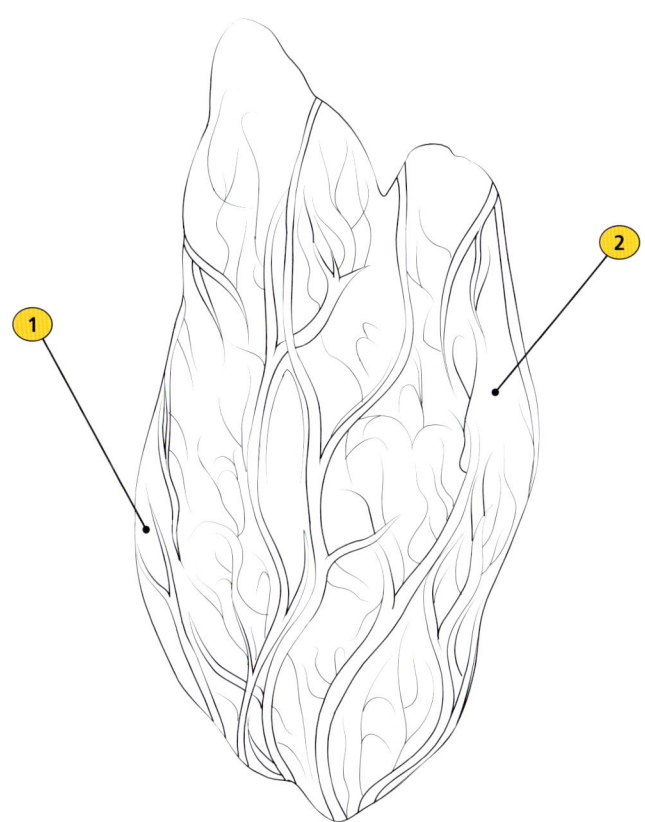

Spleen

Key:

1 Notch in superior border
2 Superior border
3 Splenic vein
4 Splenic artery (terminal branches)
5 Impression of the kidney (upper pole)
6 Impression of the colon (left colic flexure)
7 Impression of the stomach (fundus)

Description:

The spleen lies under the left ninth, tenth, and eleventh ribs, adjacent to the tail of the pancreas. Normally weighing about 5 ounces (150 g), the spleen removes particles and aged red blood cells from the bloodstream. The spleen also plays an important role in building the immune response, functioning in a similar way to lymph nodes. The organs that surround the spleen—the stomach, transverse colon, and left kidney—leave impressions on the soft surface of the spleen.

visceral surface—medial view

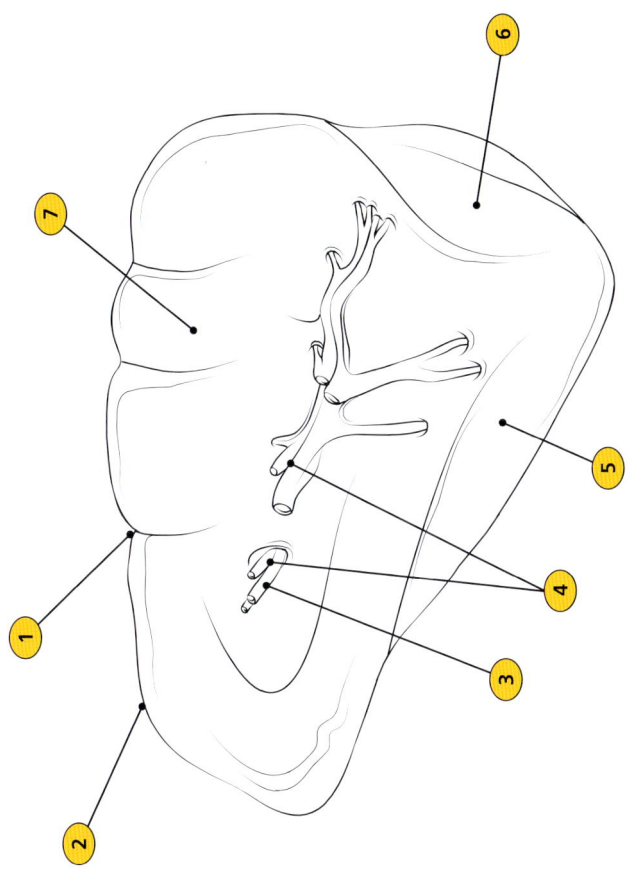

Spleen

Key:

1 Capsule
2 White pulp nodule
3 Red pulp
4 Trabecular arteries
5 Venous sinusoid

Description:

The spleen features a rich network of blood capillaries and sinusoids, called the red pulp, and aggregates of lymphocytes around branching arteries, called the white pulp.

Red blood cells are filtered through channels, called sinuses, which remove old and abnormal cells. The capillaries in the spleen are surrounded by lymphatic tissue.

microstructure

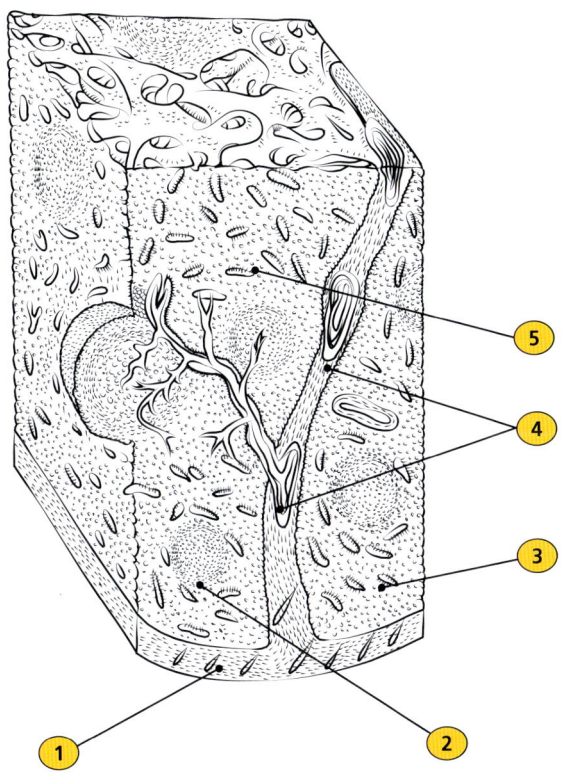

Respiratory System

The respiratory system is primarily concerned with the exchange of gases between the blood and the air of the external environment. Its primary function is therefore to bring oxygen into the lungs and the blood, and to dispose of carbon dioxide to the exterior. The respiratory system also includes the nose, which warms and moistens inhaled air and serves the sense of smell, as well as the larynx for production of the voice. The regulation of carbon dioxide by the respiratory system also helps to maintain the acid/base balance of the body.

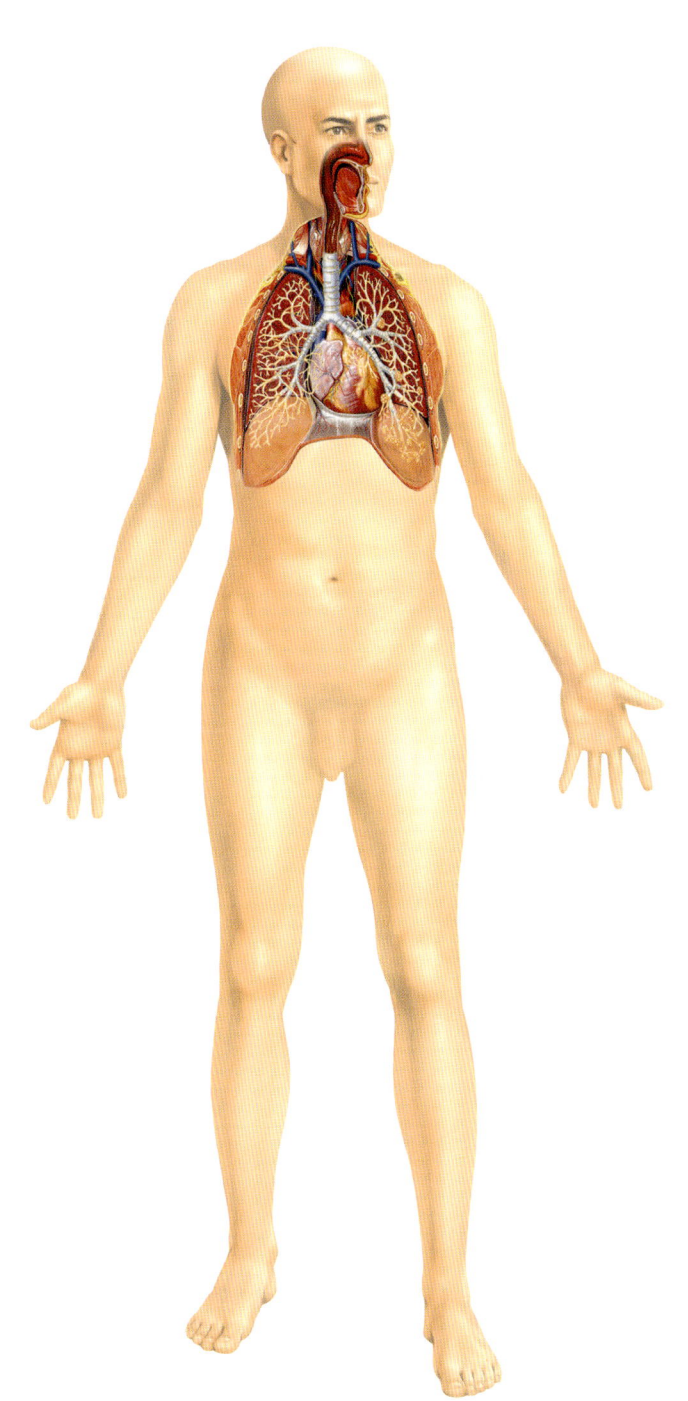

Respiratory System

Key:

1 Pharynx
2 Trachea
3 Right primary bronchus
4 Superior lobar bronchus
5 Middle lobar bronchus
6 Diaphragm
7 Left primary bronchus
8 Nasal cavity

Description:

In the process of metabolism, the body consumes oxygen and produces carbon dioxide as a waste product. The respiratory system is designed to exchange the carbon dioxide accumulated in the blood, for oxygen in the airways. The oxygen enters the lungs as air from the surrounding atmosphere via the nose, pharynx, larynx, trachea, and bronchi, and is distributed to the fine, grapelike alveoli where gas exchange can take place across a thin squamous epithelium. Ventilation of the lungs is mainly achieved by contraction of the diaphragm, which descends during inspiration, thereby expanding the vertical dimension of the chest.

Blood travels continuously through two different circulations—the systemic and the pulmonary circulations. The heart pumps deoxygenated blood from the veins of the systemic circulation into the arteries of the pulmonary circulation. This blood is oxygenated by the lungs and then flows back to the heart to be pumped into the arteries of the systemic circulation.

anterior view

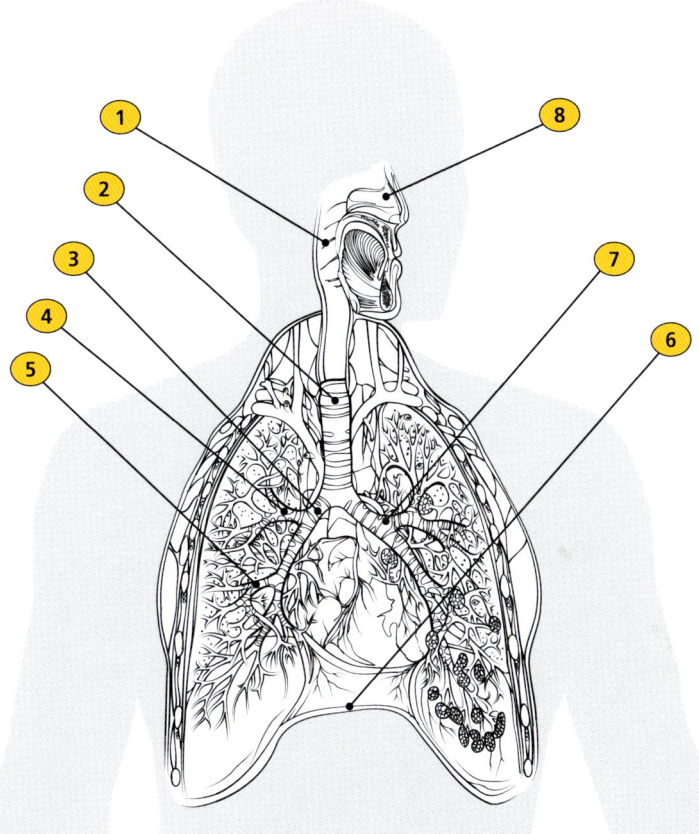

Upper Part of the Respiratory System

Key:
- **1** Nasal cavity
- **2** Nasopharynx
- **3** Oropharynx
- **4** Laryngopharynx
- **5** Larynx
- **6** Trachea

Description:

The upper part of the respiratory system consists of the nose, the nasal cavity, and the pharynx. The pharynx is divided into three parts—the nasopharynx, oropharynx, and laryngopharynx—and is shared by the respiratory and digestive systems.

The nose serves to warm and humidify inhaled air. The nostrils lead to the nasal cavities, which in turn lead to the pharynx, and then to the larynx and trachea. The nasal cavities are flattened ducts, into which protrude curved conchae (or turbinates) that increase the surface area of the nasal cavities. The nasal cavities are connected to the paranasal sinuses in the frontal, ethmoid, maxillary, and sphenoid bones of the skull. The upper part of the nasal cavity also serves the sense of smell (olfaction). The larynx guards the entrance to the lower respiratory system and also produces the sound of the voice (phonation).

sagittal view

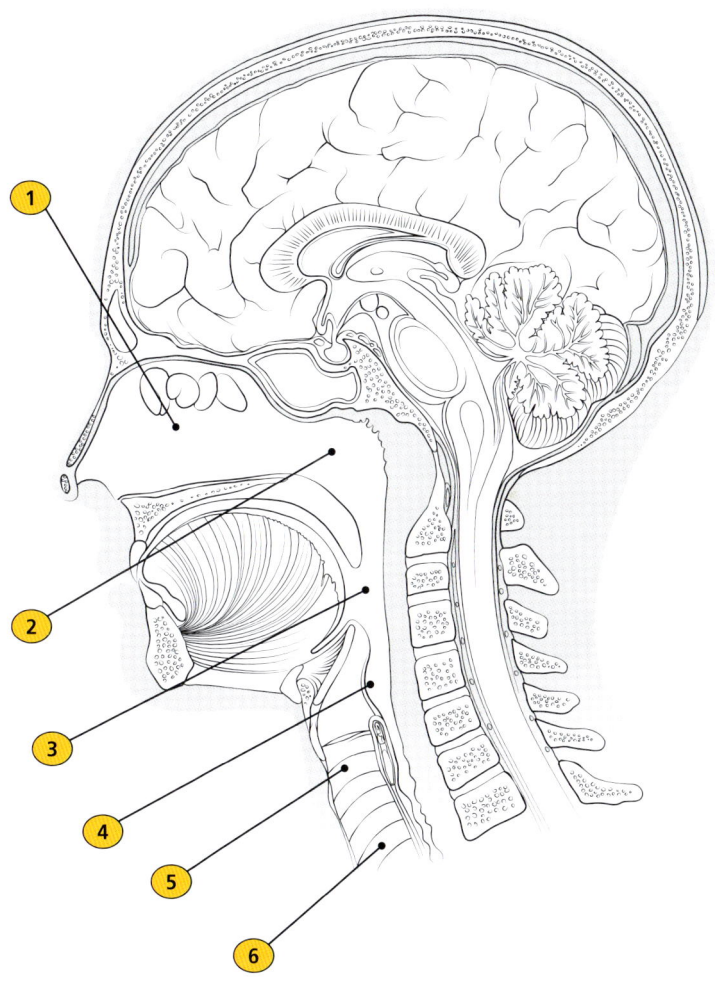

Paranasal Sinuses

Key:

1 Frontal sinus
2 Sphenoid sinus
3 Ethmoid sinus
4 Maxillary sinus

Description:

Lined with ciliated mucous membrane, the paranasal sinuses are cavities that contain air. They are situated within the frontal, sphenoid, ethmoid, and maxillary bones of the skull, and are connected by passages to the nose. The paranasal sinuses lighten the bones in which they occur, assist in cushioning blows to the head, and add resonance to the voice. The paranasal sinuses are rudimentary at birth and develop rapidly around the age of puberty.

When paranasal sinuses become filled with secretions during colds and other upper respiratory tract infections, the pressure from accumulated secretions may be felt in the various paranasal sinus regions—the frontal region (frontal sinus), the cheek (maxillary sinus), medial to the orbit (ethmoid sinuses), or deep within the head (sphenoid sinus).

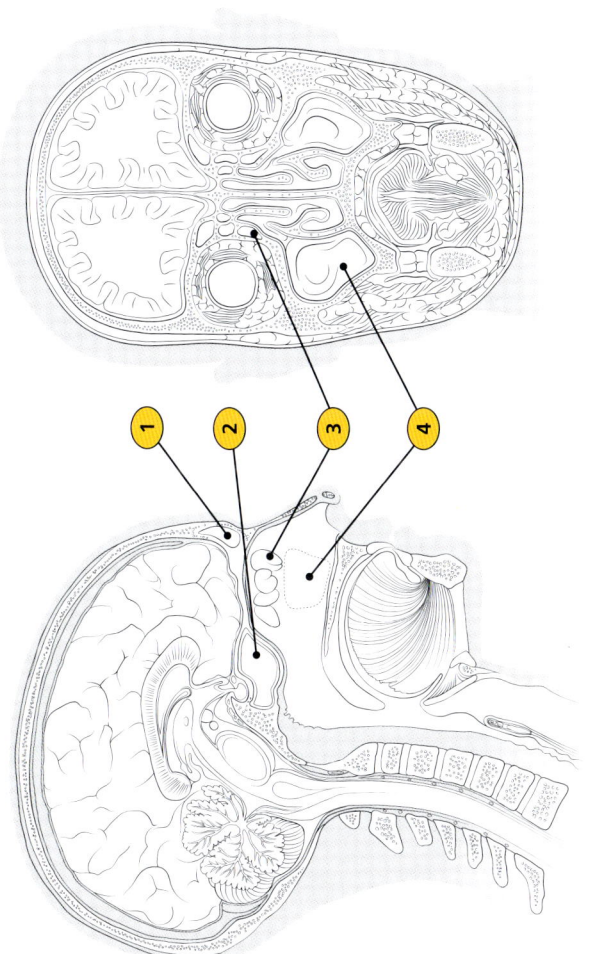

coronal view

sagittal view

Pharynx

Key:

1 Base of skull
2 Middle nasal concha
3 Inferior nasal concha
4 Soft palate
5 Uvula
6 Palatine tonsil
7 Dorsum of tongue
8 Epiglottis
9 Aryepiglottic fold
10 Esophagus
11 Parathyroid glands

12 Thyroid gland (lateral lobe)
13 Inferior constrictor muscle
14 Middle constrictor muscle
15 End of greater horn of hyoid bone
16 Stylopharyngeus muscle
17 Angle of mandible
18 Stylohyoid muscle
19 Superior constrictor muscle
20 Parotid gland

Description:

The pharynx is a common passage for air, liquid, and food. It lies behind the nasal cavity, oral cavity, and larynx, and ends in the esophagus. The pharynx comprises three parts—the nasopharynx, oropharynx, and laryngopharynx.

The nasopharynx lies immediately beneath the base of the skull and behind the nose. The nasopharynx contains tonsillar tissue in the form of the nasopharyngeal tonsils (adenoids).

The oropharynx lies behind the mouth and is separated from the mouth by paired arches of tissue on each side. The entrance from the mouth is guarded by the palatine tonsils, which lie in a fossa between the paired arches.

The laryngopharynx, or hypopharynx, is the lowest part of the pharynx and extends from the tip of the epiglottic cartilage to the lower edge of the larynx.

posterior view

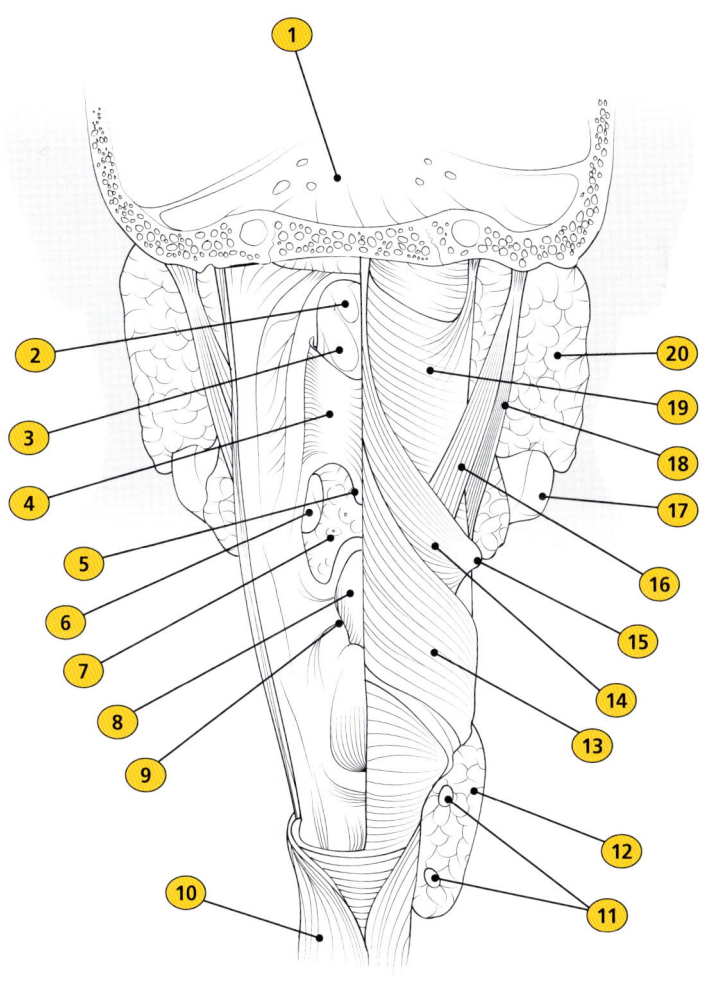

cutaway view   pharyngeal musculature

Larynx

Key:
  1 Greater horn of hyoid bone
  2 Cricothyroid muscle
  3 Tracheal cartilage
  4 Trachea
  5 Cricoid cartilage
  6 Thyroid cartilage
  7 Thyrohyoid membrane
  8 Epiglottis

Description:

The larynx extends from the back of the tongue to the trachea. The larynx is composed of nine cartilages, which provide strength for the airway and attachments for muscles, ligaments, and membranes of the larynx.

Regarded as two segments, the upper segment of the larynx commences at the epiglottis and ends at the vestibular folds or false vocal folds (false vocal cords). The lower segment begins at the vocal folds or true vocal folds (true vocal cords) and ends at the cricoid cartilage. The space between the vestibular and vocal folds is known as the ventricle of the larynx.

The cricoid cartilage is attached to the trachea below, and is the only complete ring of cartilage in the respiratory system. The vocal folds are attached to the thyroid cartilage at the front and to the arytenoid cartilages at the back. The thyroid cartilage, which is connected by a membrane to the hyoid bone above and to the cricoid cartilage below, protects the front of the larynx. The plates of the thyroid cartilage meet at a more acute angle in males (Adam's apple).

anterior view

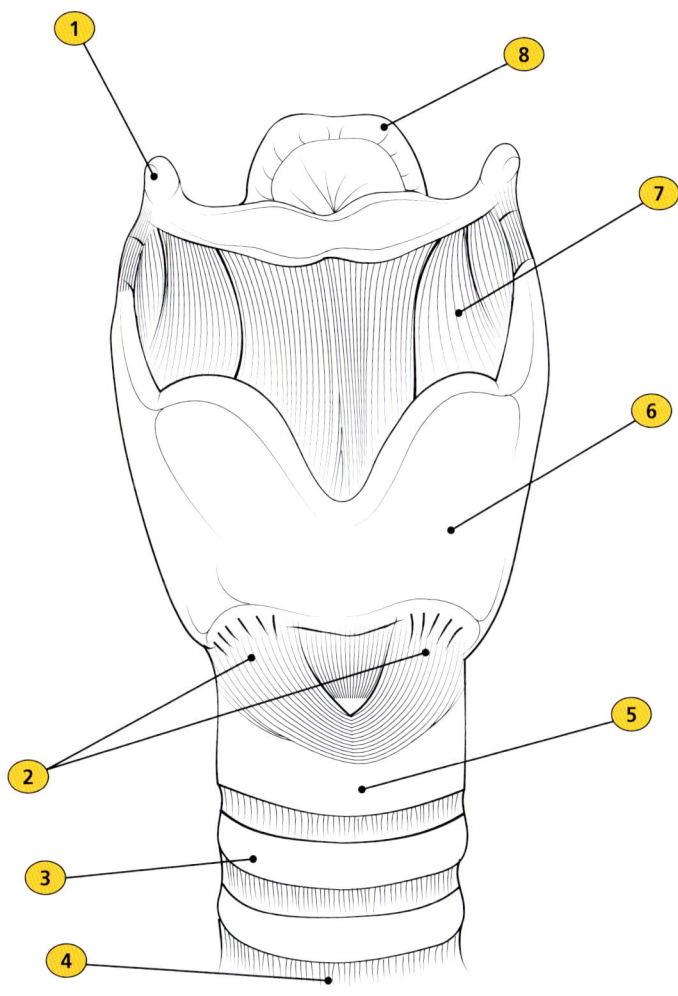

Larynx

Key:

1 Greater horn of hyoid bone
2 Superior horn of thyroid cartilage
3 Lamina of thyroid cartilage
4 Aryepiglottic fold
5 Inferior horn of thyroid cartilage
6 Capsule of cricothyroid joint
7 Tracheal cartilage
8 Trachealis muscle

9 Cricoid cartilage
10 Capsule of cricoarytenoid joint
11 Arytenoid cartilage
12 Stem of epiglottis
13 Corniculate cartilage
14 Opening for internal laryngeal nerve and vessels
15 Thyrohyoid membrane
16 Epiglottis

Description:

The larynx is a triangular box composed of nine cartilages that are joined by ligaments and controlled by skeletal muscles.

The uppermost cartilage is the epiglottis, which lies immediately behind and below the tongue and can be bent downward and backward by muscles to close off the entrance to the larynx during swallowing. The largest cartilage of the larynx, the thyroid cartilage, can be felt at the front of the throat. The thyroid cartilage is connected by a membrane to the hyoid bone above and to the cricoid cartilage, which encircles the airway, below. The other cartilages of the larynx include the arytenoids, which are paired cartilages lying on top of the cricoid cartilage, and the tiny corniculate and cuneiform cartilages, which strengthen the folds of membrane around the laryngeal entrance.

The larynx serves as a passageway for air between the pharynx and the trachea, and provides a framework for the vocal folds (vocal cords).

posterior view

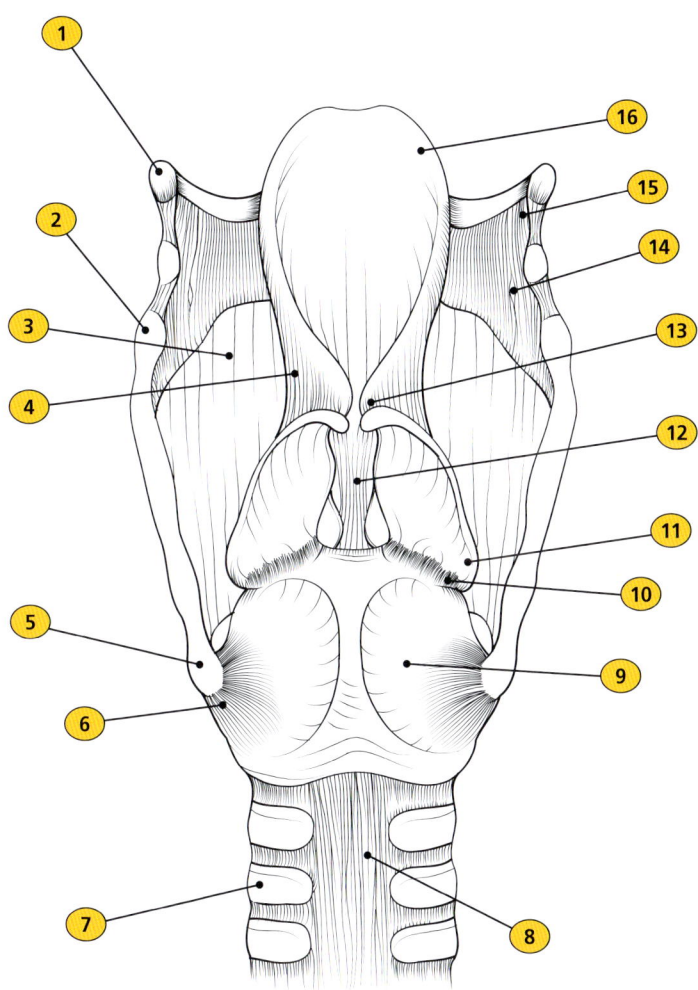

Epiglottis and Vocal Folds

Key:
1 Corniculate tubercle
2 Vocal process of arytenoid cartilage
3 View to infraglottic larynx and trachea
4 Vocal folds (vocal cords)
5 Epiglottis
6 Root of tongue

Description:

The epiglottis is a leaf-shaped flap of cartilage in the throat that lies just behind the base of the tongue and over the opening to the larynx and trachea. The vocal folds (vocal cords) consist of tent-shaped flaps of connective tissue that extend from each arytenoid cartilage posteriorly to attach to the cricoid cartilage laterally and the thyroid cartilage anteriorly. The medial free edges of the flaps—the vocal ligaments—are covered by mucous membranes to form paired vocal folds.

When the vocal folds are together and air is expelled from the lungs, this causes the vocal folds to vibrate. The arytenoid cartilages glide around a vertical axis, bringing the vocal folds closer together or further apart. The thyroid cartilage tilts on the cricoid to control the tension of the vocal folds and the frequency of the vibrations. The higher the tension, the higher the pitch of the voice. Males have longer vocal folds due to the effects of testosterone on laryngeal growth during adolescence. Longer vocal folds vibrate with a lower fundamental frequency, hence the deeper voice of males.

During inspiration, the vocal folds are separated. Air passes freely past them without making them vibrate, and so no sound is made.

superior views

laryngeal inlet closed

laryngeal inlet open—vocal folds adducted

laryngeal inlet open—vocal folds abducted

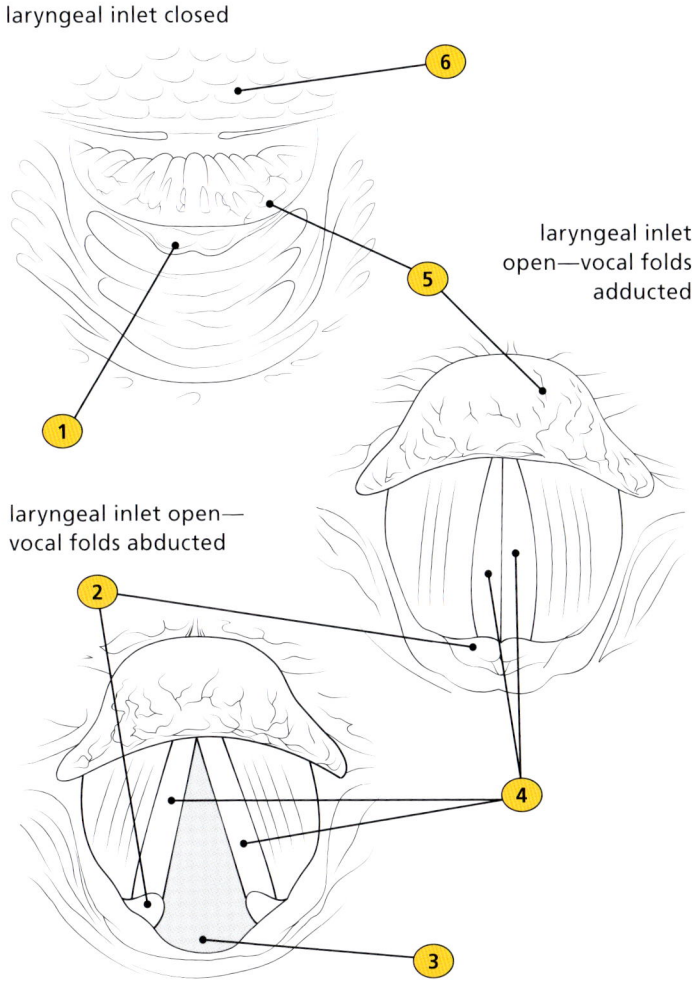

Respiratory System

Lungs and Organs of the Mediastinum

Key:

1 Brachiocephalic trunk
2 Right common carotid artery
3 Right subclavian artery
4 Right brachiocephalic vein
5 Upper lobe (right lung)
6 Ascending aorta
7 Superior vena cava
8 Transverse fissure
9 Pericardium
10 Right atrium
11 Lower lobe (right lung)
12 Visceral pleura
13 Right ventricle
14 Left ventricle
15 Pulmonary trunk
16 Left pulmonary artery
17 Left lung
18 Aortic arch
19 Left subclavian artery
20 Left common carotid artery
21 Left brachiocephalic vein

Description:

The organs of the mediastinum include the esophagus, trachea, heart, blood vessels, and thymus gland. The heart and lungs are involved in pulmonary circulation. On completion of a circuit of the body, oxygen-depleted blood is pumped by the right ventricle of the heart through the pulmonary arteries into the lungs. Branches of the pulmonary arteries follow the bronchial tree and end in the capillaries that surround the alveoli, where gas exchange occurs.

Reoxygenated blood is collected by venules that converge into two pulmonary veins for each lung, and returns to the left atrium of the heart so that it can be pumped back around the body.

The arch of the aorta has three large branches—brachiocephalic trunk, left common carotid artery, and left subclavian artery—which together supply the head and upper limbs. The aorta continues as the thoracic and abdominal aorta.

anterior view

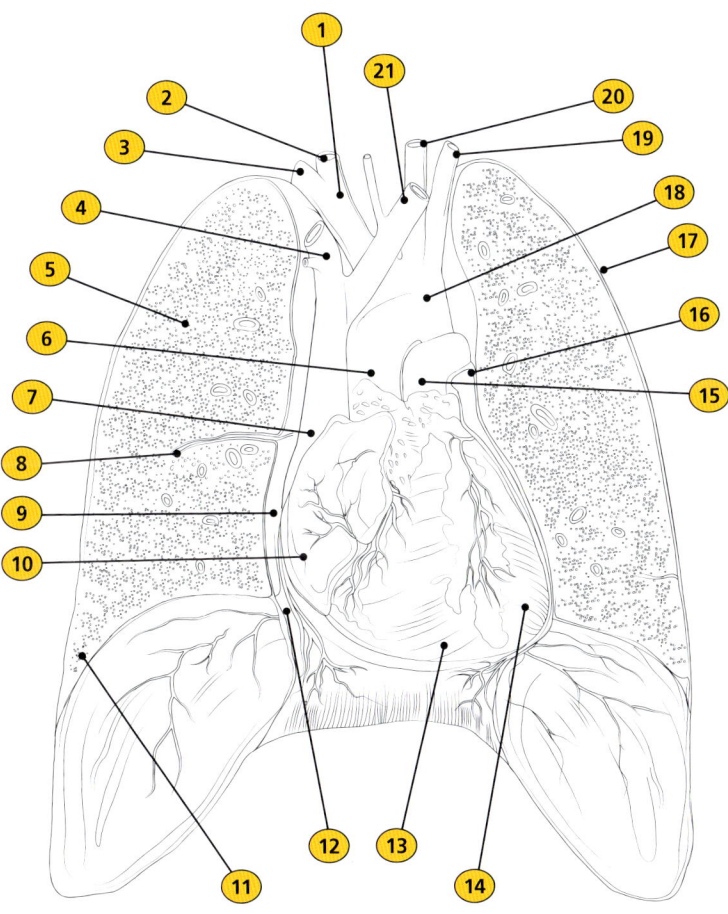

Lungs and Organs of the Mediastinum

Key:

1 Right ventricle
2 Interventricular septum
3 Left ventricle
4 Left atrium
5 Left lung
6 Rib
7 Descending aorta
8 Esophagus
9 Spinal cord

10 Body of thoracic vertebra
11 Azygos vein
12 Visceral pleura
13 Parietal pleura
14 Right lung
15 Inferior vena cava
16 Right atrium
17 Sternum

Description:

The mediastinum contains the heart, pericardium, esophagus, trachea, and associated blood vessels and nerves. The mediastinal organs are encircled by the sternum of the thoracic cage at the front, by the lungs and pleura (pleural cavities) on each side, and by the vertebral column at the back.

The mediastinum can be divided into two compartments—the superior and inferior mediastinum. The superior mediastinum is above the level of the manubriosternal joint (level of thoracic vertebra four) with the inferior mediastinum below. The inferior mediastinum may be further subdivided into three compartments—anterior, in front of the pericardial sac; middle (containing the heart, pericardium, and roots of the great vessels); and posterior (containing the esophagus, thoracic aorta, azygos vein, and assorted nerves and lymph vessels), behind the pericardial sac.

cross-sectional view from above

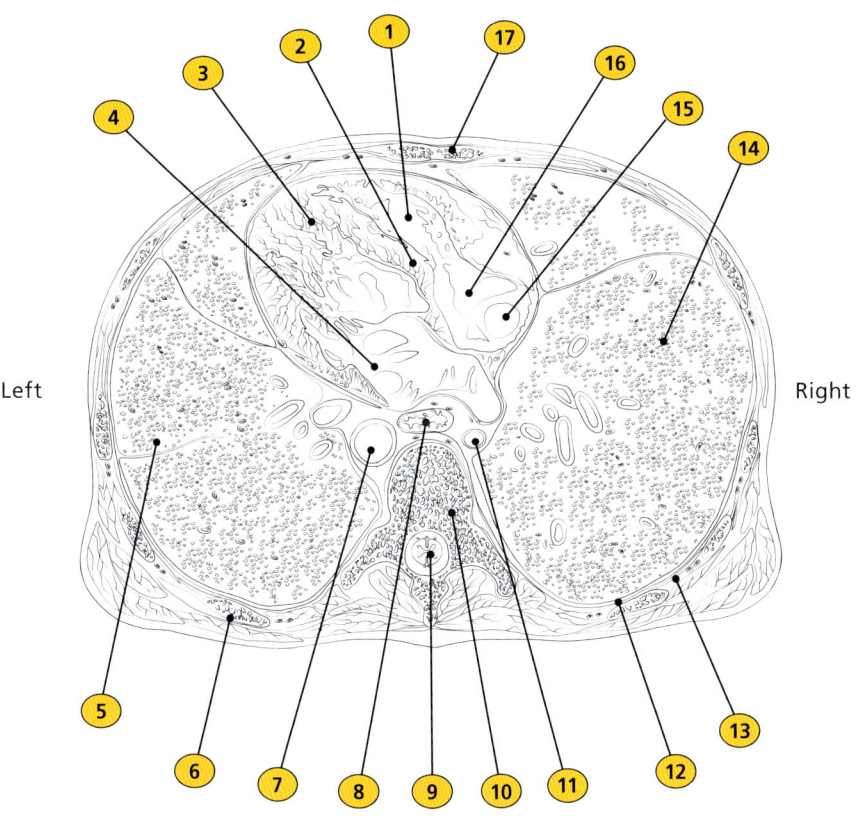

Left

Right

Lungs

Key:

1 Trachea
2 Right brachiocephalic vein
3 Thymus gland
4 Superior vena cava
5 Upper lobe (right lung)
6 Middle lobe (right lung)
7 Lower lobe (right lung)
8 Right atrium of heart
9 Right ventricle of heart
10 Pericardium
11 Diaphragm
12 Lower lobe (left lung)
13 Upper lobe (left lung)
14 Aortic arch
15 Left brachiocephalic vein
16 Internal thoracic vein
17 Vagus nerve
18 Thyroid gland (partially cut)

Description:

The lungs are the two main organs of the respiratory system, lying on either side of the heart within the chest cavity. The lungs are enclosed within pleural sacs, which provide a smooth low-friction surface that allows the lungs to move freely inside the chest. Each lung has a roughly conical or pyramidal shape, with a base sitting on top of the diaphragm; sides in contact with the rib cage (costal surface), the mediastinum (mediastinal surface), and the backbone (vertebral surface); and an apex. The lung apex is encircled by the first rib.

On the mediastinal surface of each lung is the lung hilum, where the left and right main bronchi enter the lung and the pulmonary arteries and veins enter and exit, respectively. The bronchi subdivide into the bronchioles, which in turn subdivide into the alveoli.

The lungs are divided into lobes—usually three in the right lung and two in the left lung—by a series of clefts or fissures. A horizontal or transverse fissure is usually found in the right lung and oblique fissures in both the left and right lungs.

anterior view

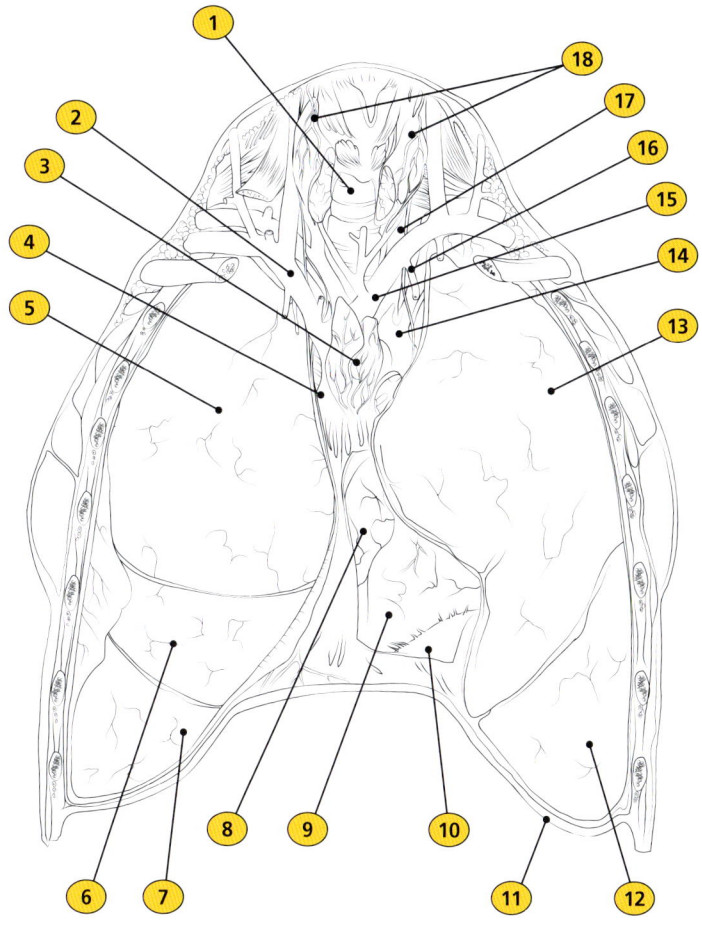

Trachea and Bronchi in situ

Key:
1 Trachea
2 Right main (primary) bronchus
3 Superior lobar bronchi
4 Middle lobar bronchus
5 Inferior lobar bronchi
6 Right lung
7 Left lung
8 Left main (primary) bronchus

Description:

The trachea is a 3½–5 inch (9–12.5 cm) long and ⅗ inch (1.5 cm) wide tube for the passage of air. It begins at the lower end of the larynx and passes into the thoracic cavity, where it terminates by dividing into the left and right main (primary) bronchi.

The trachea is a fibroelastic and muscular structure, reinforced by 15–20 C-shaped cartilages connected to each other by fibrous tissue. The cartilages prevent the collapse of the airway, and the elastic fibers allow it to stretch and recoil with the movement of the larynx and diaphragm. The back of the trachea is flat. Here, the ends of the cartilage are bridged by the transversely oriented trachealis muscle, whose contractions reduce the diameter of the airway. The esophagus lies against this surface and expands into the gap in the cartilage during swallowing. The trachea is lined with mucous membrane, and the cilia in the membrane serve to move dust-laden particles toward the throat for elimination.

The right main (primary) bronchus is usually a little wider and more vertical than the left and, therefore, is more often the site of impaction of inhaled foreign bodies (for example, peanuts).

anterior view

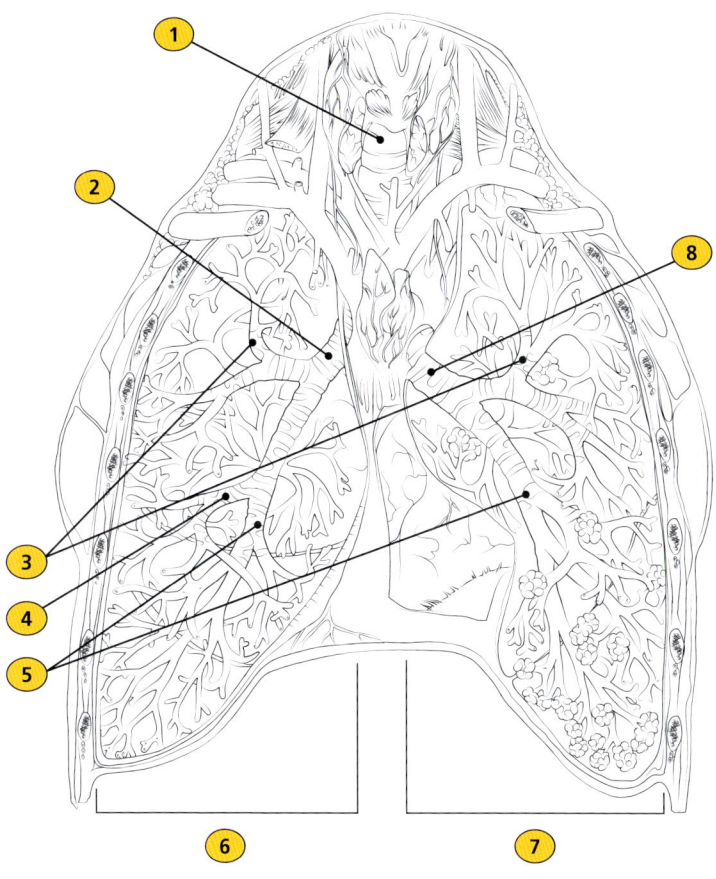

Trachea

Key:
1 Cartilage
2 Submucosal gland
3 Trachealis muscle
4 Annular ligament
5 Respiratory epithelium

Description:
The structural elements of the trachea are shown in this cross-section. The trachea is reinforced at the front and sides by C-shaped plates of cartilage, which keep the passageway open. Bridging the ends of the cartilage is the trachealis muscle, which is governed by the autonomic nervous system, and serves to alter the diameter of the trachea.

The internal lining of the trachea is respiratory epithelium, which overlies a layer of connective tissue called the lamina propria. These two layers form the respiratory mucosa, beneath which lies the submucosa that contains the submucosal glands.

The posterior wall of the trachea is soft to accommodate the expansion of the esophagus when swallowing. This is especially important at the level of the thoracic inlet (encircled by the first rib), where many structures—trachea, esophagus, common carotid arteries, jugular veins—pass through a confined space.

cross-sectional view

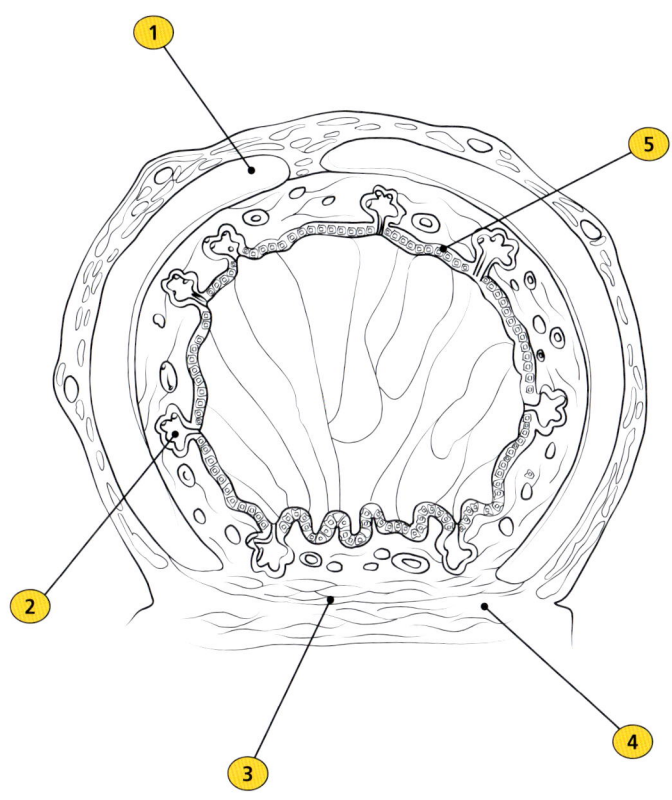

Bronchial Tree

Key:

1 Trachea
2 Right main (primary) bronchus
3 Secondary bronchi
4 Tertiary bronchi

5 Bronchioles
6 Alveoli
7 Left main (primary) bronchus

Description:

At its lower end, the trachea branches into the right main (primary) bronchus, which leads to the right lung, and the left main (primary) bronchus, which serves the left lung. The route from the trachea through the right main bronchus is more vertical, wider, and shorter than it is to the left.

The wall of each bronchus is supported by cartilage. The C-shaped cartilage is bridged by the trachealis muscle to complete the tubular formation of the bronchus. The interior is lined with mucous membrane and many microscopic, mobile, hairlike cilia.

The main bronchus branches into smaller secondary bronchi at the lung's entrance. These are also called lobar bronchi, because one of them serves each lung lobe. Each secondary bronchus divides into smaller tertiary bronchi. These bronchi split into subsequent generations of smaller and smaller bronchi, which finally split into bronchioles that separate into terminal bronchioles—the bronchioles are entirely muscular and have no cartilage in their walls. The bronchioles end at the microscopic air sacs (alveoli), where the exchange of carbon dioxide for oxygen occurs. Alveoli are separated from one another by interalveolar septa, which greatly increase the surface area for gas exchange. Lying on the inner surface of the alveolar walls are macrophages, which engulf inhaled bacteria, dust, or carbon particles.

anterior view

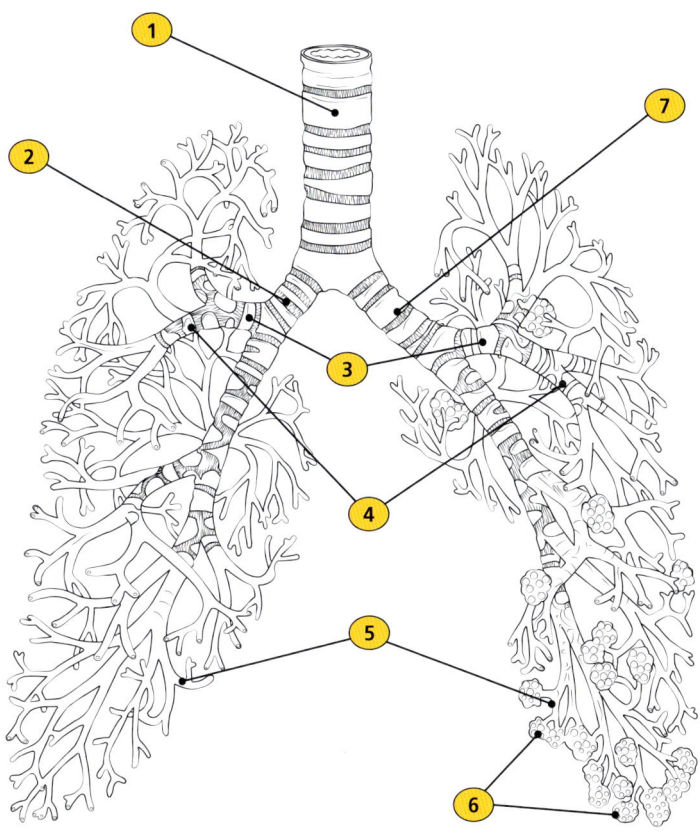

Bronchus

Key:

1 Submucosa
2 Smooth muscle
3 Respiratory epithelium
4 Submucosal gland
5 Cartilage

Description:

Similar in composition to the trachea, the bronchi and bronchioles feature a muscular exterior, and are internally lined with respiratory epithelium. Cartilage also forms part of the structure of bronchi, but as the bronchi subdivide, the amount of cartilage gradually lessens, and when the bronchioles are reached, there is no cartilage present.

The respiratory epithelium of the bronchi overlies a layer of lamina propria and a submucosal layer. Within the submucosal layer are submucosal glands. The bronchial lining also features cilia, which, in combination with the submucosal glands, ensure that the bronchial airways remain clear. The bronchial lining also contains lymphoid tissue because the respiratory system is constantly exposed to foreign proteins and microorganisms.

cross-sectional view

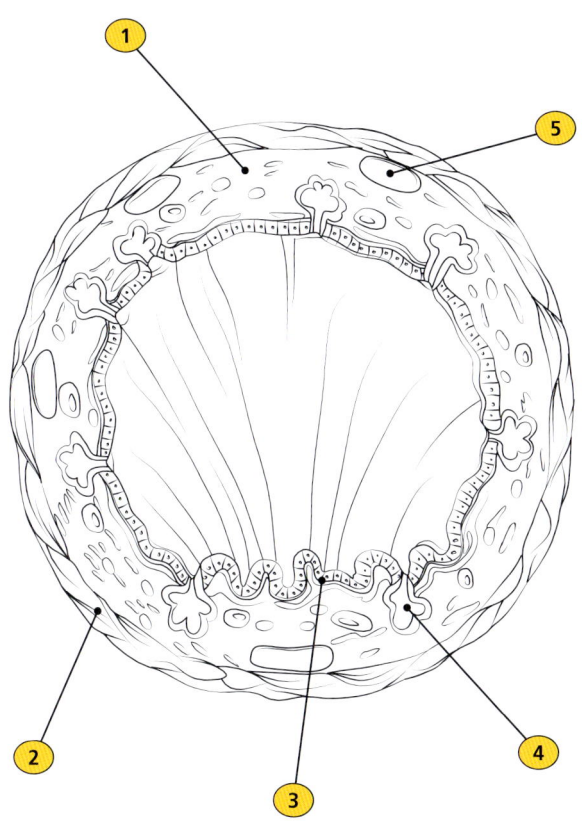

Respiratory Muscles: Intercostal Muscles

Key:
1 Manubrium of the sternum
2 Body of sternum
3 Costal cartilage
4 Xiphoid process
5 Rectus abdominus muscle
6 External intercostal muscles
7 Internal intercostal muscles
8 Ribs 8–10 (floating ribs)
9 Ribs 1–7 (true ribs)
10 Sternoclavicular joint

Description:
The internal and external intercostal muscles connecting the ribs, in conjunction with the diaphragm, are the primary muscles involved in executing the movements required to increase the capacity of the thoracic cage. The obliquely arranged intercostal muscles bridge between, and move, neighboring ribs, connecting the inferior border of the upper rib to the superior border of the rib below. When air is breathed in (inspiration), the ribs move around their vertebral articulations, and the sternum connected to the true ribs is elevated, thus raising the ribs. Although inspiration is mostly due to the contraction of the diaphragm, the intercostal muscles do make a contribution, particularly during exercise or disease.

Expiration is a passive process—the muscles of the thoracic cage recoil to their resting position, returning the thoracic cage to its original size, and pushing air from the lungs as a result.

anterior view

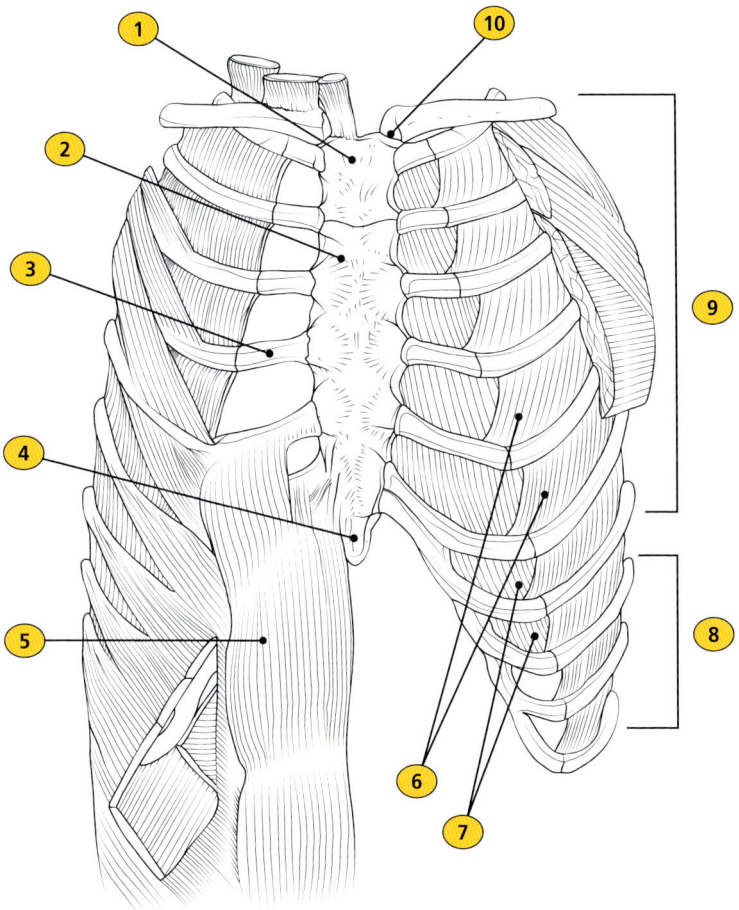

Respiratory Muscles: Diaphragm

Key:

1 Body of sternum
2 Xiphoid process
3 Inferior vena cava
4 Central tendon
5 Twelfth rib
6 Celiac trunk
7 Abdominal aorta
8 Right crus of diaphragm
9 Vertebral column
10 Left crus of diaphragm
11 Quadratus lumborum muscle
12 Esophagus

Description:

The diaphragm is the muscular layer that separates the chest cavity from the abdominal cavity. Along with the intercostal muscles, it is one of the principal muscles used in respiration. When the diaphragm is at rest, it forms a high dome; when the diaphragm contracts, this dome descends, thus increasing the height of the thoracic cavity. Increasing the height of the thoracic cavity in turn draws air into the lungs. Expiration is a passive process—occurring as a result of relaxation of tension in the soft and hard tissues of the chest and abdomen.

The diaphragm is perforated by three large openings—the aortic hiatus, the inferior vena caval hiatus, and the esophageal hiatus.

inferior view

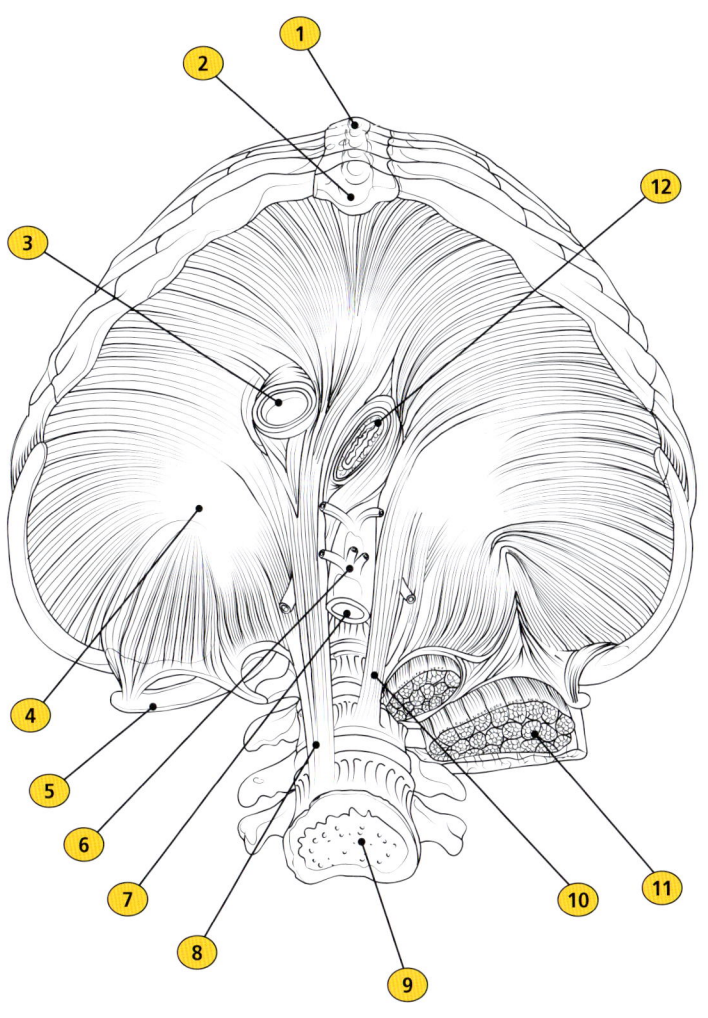

Index

Index